IN THE
FOOTSTEPS
OF THE
YELLOW EMPEROR:

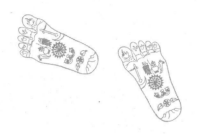

TRACING
THE HISTORY OF
TRADITIONAL ACUPUNCTURE

by Peter Eckman, M.D., Ph.D., M.Ac. (UK)

CYPRESS BOOK COMPANY
SAN FRANCISCO

IN THE FOOTSTEPS OF THE YELLOW EMPEROR:

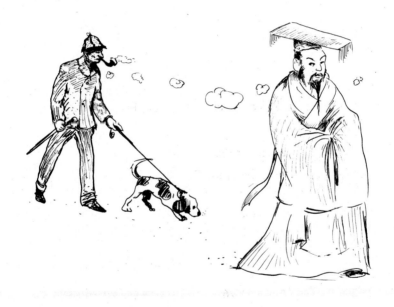

TRACING THE HISTORY OF TRADITIONAL ACUPUNCTURE

Dedicated to
Yanagiya Sorei and Tobe Soshichiro* —

whose lives embodied not just the letter,
but the very spirit of traditional Oriental medicine;

whose work helped build the bridge between
East and West
across which I invite you to travel with me.

* With a special "thank you" to
Chieko Maekawa
for being my go-between.

TABLE OF CONTENTS

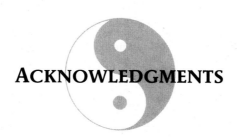

ACKNOWLEDGMENTS

My heartfelt thanks to the following individuals who allowed me to informally "interview" them — in person, by telephone or through correspondence: John Amaro, Kenneth Basham, Dan Bensky, Stephen Birch, Johannes Bischko, August Brodde, Vivienne Brown, the late Harry Cadman, Cai Jingfeng, Ursula Cantieni (stepdaughter of the late Heribert Schmidt), Cao Guoliang, Pedro Chan, Mme. Veuve Chamfrault (wife of the late Albert Chamfault), Cecil Chen, Alan Covell, Jon Covell, Ralph Dale, John D'Ambrosio, Jacques De Langre, Luc De Schepper, Mark Drue, William Dufty, Bob Duggan, Jean-Marc Eyssalet, Tony Evans, Gerald Fabian, Peter Firebrace, Galen Fisher, Bob Flaws, the late Geoff Foulkes, his wife Gillian Foulkes, Charles Fox, Fukushima Kodo, Robert Gerzon, Joseph Goodman, Claude Grégory, Gérard Guillaume, Hashimoto Mariko (granddaughter of the late Hashimoto Masae), Joe Helms, Margaret Ho (daughter of the late Hsu Mifoo), John Hsu (son of the late Hsu Mifoo), Anton Jayasuriya, Eric W. Johnson, Ted Kaptchuk, Jean-Marc Kespi, Ronald Kotzsch, Kuon Dowon, Michio Kushi, Stuart Kutchins, Keith Lamont, Roger Langrick, Claude Larre, the late Jacques Lavier, his daughter Marie-Christine Lavier, the late Denis Lawson-Wood, his wife Joyce Lawson-Wood, Miriam Lee, Paul Lepron, Leung Kok-Yuen, the late Li Zhi-sui, Liang Shen-ping, Luying Liaw, Lok Yee-Kung, Royston Low, Ralph Luciani, Chieko Maekawa, Felix Mann, Bryan Manuele, David Marks, Julia Measures, Barbara Mitchell, In Moon, Maurice Mussat, Nagayama Toyoko (wife of the late Nagayama Kunzo), Diane Nathan, Roger Newman-Turner, Jean Niboyet-fils (son of the late Jean Niboyet), Edward Obaidey, Hiroshisa Oda, Ono Bunkei (via his daughter), William Peacher, Rolla Pennell, Manfred Porkert, Qiu Mao-liang, Ren Jianning, Yves Réquéna, the late James Reston and his wife Sally Reston, Françoise Rivière, Miles Roberts, his wife Chie Roberts, Sidney and Pat Rose-Neil, Michael Rosoff, Mme. J. Schatz (wife of the late Jean Schatz), K.M. Schipper, the late Heribert Schmidt, Claus Schnorrenberger, Mark Seem, George Serres, Miki Shima, Jim Shores, Shudo Denmei, Siow Yong-Chai, Hillary Skellon (daughter of J.R. Worsley), Nicholas Sofroniou, Sorimachi Taiichi, Malcolm Stemp, Frank Sun, Takenouchi Misao, Eric Tao, Bill Tara, Tashima Sensei, Radha Thambirajah, Tobe Soshichiro, Angela Tu, Paul Unschuld, J.D. Van Buren, Marc Van Cauwenberghe, Nguyen Van Nghi, Solange Voiret, Stuart Watts, Mario Wexu, Allegra Wint, Henry Wong, Louise Wong (niece of the late Hsu Mifoo), J.R. Worsley, John Worsley (son of J.R. Worsley),

William Wright, Wu Wei-p'ing, Shinichiro Yamada, Shizuko Yamamoto, Yanagiya Masako (second wife of the late Yanagiya Sorei) Richard Yennie, Clim Yoshimi, Jeffrey Yuen, and Zeng Guoyuan. My apologies to anyone I've inadvertantly left out — in a work such as this one, I fear it must be inevitable.

Some of the source material I used is in foreign languages. I am indebted to the following individuals for their translational assistance: Chieko Maekawa – Japanese, Luying Liaw – Chinese, Hai-ja Lew – Korean, Klaus Maaser and Linda Dvornik – German, Joe Helms – French. I have indicated in the text whenever I attempted translations on my own.

Thanks to Judy Cohen for doing all the typing; to Stuart Kutchins for the countless hours of schmoozing during which most of the philosophical issues I discuss first became crystallized; to Neal White for his inimitable drawings, photographic expertise and unflagging editorial encouragement; to Dean Lander and John Worsley for the graphic and moral support of the College of Traditional Acupuncture, U.K.; and to Bob Duggan of the Traditional Acupuncture Institute whom I've always (privately) regarded as an ace up my sleeve. I also owe a heavy debt of gratitude to Zhang Xiao-jiang of Cypress Books for seeing to it that my work might reach a wider public than my small circle of friends — he is truly the good fairy who made this dream come true, with the able assistance of Linda Revel—in the graphics and Foster Stockwell who compiled the index.

Last, but not least, I wish to thank my family for sharing me with my muse. My wife Claire's aesthetic sense has been a reliable anchor, but it is her love and that of our children, Chris and Noelle, that has been my fuel.

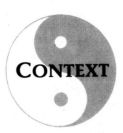

CONTEXT

Acupuncture is the practice of inserting needles into the body to activate a change in its state of functioning. There are many ways of using acupuncture, perhaps the most well-known being its spectacular ability to substitute for conventional anaesthesia, in allowing major surgery to be carried out on awake and cooperative patients, without their experiencing any pain or suffering. This procedure is called acupuncture analgesia, and was developed in China in the 1950's (Fig.1).

Thousands of years before that, in the same part of the world, acupuncture was used to treat and prevent disease and other disorders of the human organism. It developed there as part of the indigenous health care system called traditional Oriental medicine. This use of acupuncture is therefore called traditional acupuncture (Fig.2).

This book is about the history of traditional acupuncture, the culture in which it developed, and its migration West.

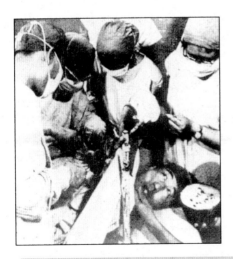
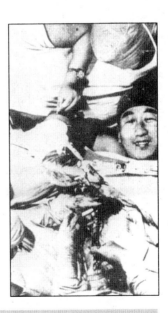

Figure 1: ACUPUNCTURE ANALGESIA.
This patient is undergoing an open-lung operation in Beijing with acupuncture as the only "anaesthetic." The two views show the patient smiling and eating watermelon during surgery!

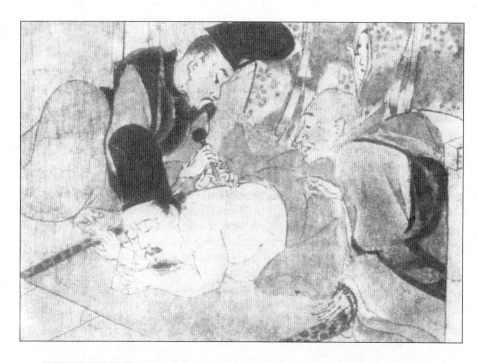

Figure 2: TRADITIONAL ACUPUNCTURE.

There are many styles of acupuncture that have developed in a traditional context. This painting depicts a Japanese approach in which a guide tube is used to insert the needle. The practitioner's concentration and concern for the patient's well-being are evident.

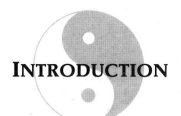

INTRODUCTION

There have been three seminal events that catalyzed the tremendous popularity of acupuncture and Oriental medicine in the U.S. in the latter half of the twentieth century. The first two were President Nixon's visit to the People's Republic of China in 1972 following shortly after the successful acupuncture treatment for post-operative pain of *New York Times* reporter James Reston in Beijing. Nixon's overture to China bespoke an about-face on the part of the previously belligerent power elite towards this communist giant, while Reston's experience had a serious impact on the media and the intellectual community, which together may be as influential a force in modern America as the power structure's infamous military-industrial complex. The third event was the publication in 1983 of Ted Kaptchuk's best-selling book, *The Web That Has No Weaver—Understanding Chinese Medicine,*[1] a work that for the first time explained many of the principles of Chinese medicine in a personal style that began to affect a much larger segment of the American populace, one which was already in the midst of a period of questioning the monopoly on health care of conventional Western medicine. What ties the affairs of Nixon, Reston and Kaptchuk together in the context of the story you are about to read, is that the image they project of Chinese medicine is that of a well-defined, homogeneous, almost monolithic discipline.

It is curious that no thorough historical account of the development of this popular style of Chinese medicine has as yet been written, at least in English. Were such a history to be documented, I believe it would show that Traditional Chinese Medicine, this officially approved methodology which is promoted by the Chinese government, and which I will henceforth refer to as TCM, was itself a creation of the latter half of the twentieth century, and is in fact only one line of development among many from a conglomeration of theories and practices in the Orient stretching back to the stone age, and which I will refer to by the more generic and inclusive label, traditional Oriental medicine, or TOM.

During the same time that TCM and its style of acupuncture were becoming popular in the West, other styles of acupuncture were emerging from the mother discipline, TOM. As early as the 1930's, these other styles, reflecting practices in Japan, Korea, Vietnam and other Oriental countries, also began to migrate West, and had their initial impact on Europe.[2] A cross-fertilization occurred, as it will whenever two cultures come into contact, and European acupuncture began to incorporate some of the Western vitalistic ideas which were cognate with the basic theories of TOM, while in China, the influence of Western medical thinking on the nascent TCM was a substantial one, as was also the case in Japan and Korea.

The outcome of this process of historical development is that contrary to popular thought, there are currently many distinct styles of acupuncture, each of which can be considered traditional insofar as it has evolved from the common progenitor, TOM, and honors its original root (Fig.3).

It would not be feasible for me to trace in equal detail the evolution of each of these unique styles of acupuncture. For reasons I will explain shortly, I have chosen one particular style, Leamington Acupuncture, which I will henceforth refer to as LA, to be the focus of this historical study. LA,

TRADITIONAL (based mainly on TOM paradigms)	NON-TRADITIONAL (based on non-TOM paradigms)	MIXED (based on a combination of TOM & non-TOM paradigms)
Traditional Chinese Medicine- TCM (China)	Auriculotherapy (France)	Ryodoraku (Japan)
Tong Family Style (Taiwan)		Electroacupuncture According to Voll- EAV (Germany)
Eight Constitutions (Korea)		New Acupuncture (China)
Meridian Therapy - MT (Japan)		
Six Energetic Levels (France)		
Leamington Acupuncture - LA (England)		

Figure 3: VARIOUS STYLES OF ACUPUNCTURE THERAPY
Although all of these uses of acupuncture have demonstrated their clinical efficacy, this historical study is restricted to the traditional styles, and in particular focuses on the last entry LA, and contrasts it with TCM, the first entry.

like TCM, represents a style of acupuncture which developed in the twentieth century based on ancient principles and is widely practiced in the United States and Great Britain. It is more commonly known as Five Element acupuncture, after its main guiding theory. TCM on the other hand, is based on a different paradigm, the Eight Principles for Differentiating Syndromes, for which reason its style of practice is popularly referred to as Eight Principle acupuncture. For the benefit of the reader who may not be familiar with these terms, or the other technical material to which I will refer in the historical narrative, I have included two preliminary chapters as an acupuncture primer of sorts. I would like this book to be accessible to the lay reader, while still maintaining its appeal to those in the profession itself. Thus, some of this material may seem either overly technical or too elementary, but I would encourage the reader to persevere through these passages as I have included them for the sake of referencing important material to be introduced later on. Following the didactic section I will begin my tale with a look at ancient China through its mythology so as to recreate the setting in which acupuncture first developed. Then I will trace acupuncture's historical origin and evolution, first in Asia and finally in the West.

Admittedly, all of what follows is written from a decidedly subjective point of view formed by twenty years in the study and practice of TOM so perhaps I should begin first with a little personal history. My initial training was in Western medicine and physiology, and it was only afterwards, in 1973, that I began to study acupuncture under Kim Se Han , a Korean practitioner living in Los Angeles. My exposure to acupuncture and the panoply of teachings which make up TOM was a transformative experience that determined the future course of my professional career. I subsequently began studying with Professor J.R. Worsley of the College of Traditional Acupuncture in Leamington Spa, England, and was somewhat shocked to discover that the Five Element style which he teaches is quite different from the Korean style I had begun learning; and both of these styles were different, yet again, from TCM which I later studied in China. By the time I was exposed to Japanese and Vietnamese styles of acupuncture I was no longer shocked by their differences, but rather eager to discover the unique teachings of each and how they could help shed further light on the nature of human life in health and in illness, which is the essence of TOM.

In my experience, all of the varieties of acupuncture which I have investigated have proved to be powerful and at times miraculous tools for health care when used by well-trained practitioners. My training in England left me however, with a particular fascination regarding the style of practice taught by Professor Worsley (Fig.4). His approach specifically aims at touching the more intimate levels of human experience, especially the life of the Spirit which was one of the original foundations of TOM. Worsley's style

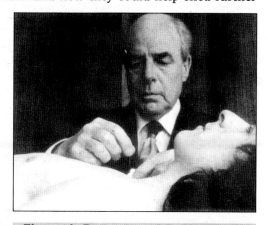

Figure 4: PROFESSOR J.R. WORSLEY.
Although Professor Worsley doesn't use a guide tube to insert needles, his level of concentration and concern as an acupuncture practitioner is reminiscent of the medieval Japanese practitioner in Figure 2.

has come to be known as Leamington Acupuncture or LA after the location of the main school where it is taught. The history of LA is even less well-documented then that of TCM, to which I will be comparing it, and has led to insinuations that LA, far from being traditional, was purely a creation of Worsley himself. Certainly, there have been understandable requests for some historical documentation.[3]

Which brings me to an explanation of how I came to write this book. It was only on a recent lecture trip to England that I was labelled as being an historian. For the past twenty years I have thought of myself first as a physician, and foremost as an acupuncturist, but now that I think about it, I have been doing historical fieldwork for just about as long as anything else. My dear friend Allegra Wint from Oxford reminded me of a dinner party some of us students gave for Professor Worsley when we were beginning our acupuncture studies with him back in 1974. While my classmates took it upon themselves to make it a social evening, I used the occasion to pester my revered teacher with questions about his background—where did he learn such-and-such, did he study with so-and-so, etc? Perhaps the reason I became something of an historian was due to his persistent reticence. As I didn't get much information out of him, I just kept asking the same questions over and over again of anyone who might have some information, until it became a part of me—a quest, or perhaps simply a Zen koan. In any case, this process reflects the focus of my discussion of Western acupuncture on Worsley and LA. In no way do I wish to imply that the other styles of acupuncture taught in the West, even in England itself, are any less authentic. In fact, I will discuss many of them in passing, but as my process in this regard has been the attempt to shed light on the mystery of where Worsley got his goods, I have reported the results of my detective work as they materialized from the numerous letters sent and interviews conducted around the world over the years.

On a similar note, my choice of TCM as the "foil"—that is, as the dominant style of acupuncture with which to contrast the teachings of LA is not meant as a slight to any of the other styles of acupuncture practiced in the Orient. The dedication of this book reflects the debt of gratitude I feel to the Japanese tradition, both for the historical role it has played and for the assistance its practitioners provided in gathering the necessary materials to tell this story. I wish in doing my research I could have used the same method of interviews and letters for tracing the development of TCM—unfortunately I have had neither the time, the contacts, nor the linguistic skills to do a proper job of it, so my account therefore is based entirely on secondary sources. Finally, my capsule presentation of the long history of TOM is admittedly far from complete, and is offered simply as an ice-breaker. If my work turns out to be somewhat amusing and educational without being too offensive to the established professors of history, then its purpose will have been fulfilled.

I might jump the gun here with a bit of contemporary history which I think nicely illustrates some of the themes I will be discussing. Let's go back to July 12, 1971, when the aforementioned James Reston finally arrived in Beijing after having been delayed in his trip from the U.S. for several days in Canton by bureaucratic red tape. He was anxious to interview the Chinese leadership in the capital, which would have been quite a reportorial coupe as China had, until then, been closed behind a "bamboo curtain" for quite some time. You can imagine, then, his reaction when he was informed on his arrival in Beijing that Henry Kissinger had just "scooped" him by announcing plans for President Nixon to pay an official visit to China the following year (Fig.5). As soon as this news was delivered, Reston felt a sharp pain in his abdomen which developed into a classical case of

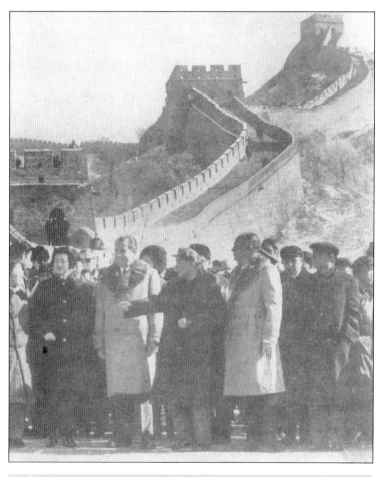

Figure 5: RICHARD NIXON IN CHINA
Nixon's ceremonial visit to the Great Wall took place in 1972.

appendicitis. He was rushed to the Anti-Imperialist Hospital (which by the way, was formerly the Peking Union Medical College, built and paid for by the Rockefeller Foundation in 1916) where he underwent an emergency appendectomy under conventional Western anaesthesia. In the following days, he began to experience post-operative abdominal pain and distention and was offered acupuncture as a possible treatment. This was accepted, and he was treated by the staff acupuncturist who inserted three needles in his right elbow and below his knees, and then used burning moxa[4] to warm his abdomen. This treatment was successful in relieving his distress, and the Western world began to hear about acupuncture in a big way (Fig.6). Now Reston's treatment serves as a good example of the practice of TCM—his condition was handled as an organic physiological derangement, both from the point of view of Western medicine and of TCM which were used conjointly to successfully treat him. But what of Reston's own perception of the experience? He was quite clear that the most sensible explanation for his illness was his reaction to the news of Kissinger's triumph. The relationship of the mind and the body has become a prominent field of study which in the context of health care has led to the development of "psychosomatic medicine." Curiously enough, it is just this psychosomatic

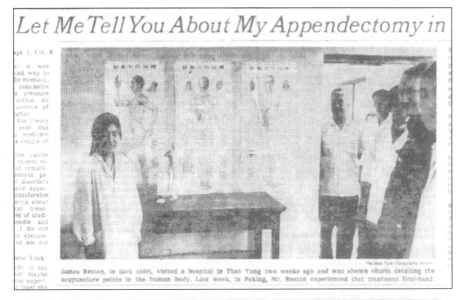

Figure 6: JAMES RESTON IN CHINA.
Following his recuperation from surgery, Reston was photographed visiting the acupuncture department of a hospital in Thao Yang, and he was instrumental in exposing many Westerners to acupuncture for the first time.

approach, in which terms Reston tried to understand his illness, which is the primary focus of LA. Thus, in addition to addressing Reston's abdominal discomfort, an acupuncturist of the LA persuasion would have tried to ensure that Reston's troubled Spirit had also been eased, using needles and moxa for instruments, just as had the TCM acupuncturist. In this anecdote I am caricaturing TCM and LA more or less in the following ways: I see TCM as having adopted those elements of TOM that are most compatible with Western science. The thrust of its development has indeed been to integrate these two materialist approaches to health care so that its practitioners might most appropriately be referred to as doctors. LA on the other hand, seems to me to have preferentially adopted those elements of TOM of a more metaphysical character: the place of Man in the cosmos, and the meaning—be it physical, psychological or spiritual—of his moment to moment experience in health or in illness which assigns its practitioners to a role that might better be termed "healer" or "medicine man." In order to understand how these different styles of "traditional acupuncture" compare, and how each of them can stand as complete systems of medicine parallel to the one we are familiar with in the West, I have developed a model which I will elaborate in the first two chapters, following which we will travel backwards in time several thousand years in an attempt to discover the origins of these arcane practices.

The Circle

It is impossible to write an intelligent history of traditional acupuncture without establishing at least a basic level of understanding of the subject matter itself. There are several books that I think do a good job and which I encourage the reader to investigate for some alternative points of view, but I cannot avoid the necessity of covering this ground myself.[5]

Acupuncture simply means the insertion of needles into the body to bring about some desired change as a result of the needles' direct effects, and not from the injection of any materials through the needle. There are many ways to use needles to produce acupunctural effects as illustrated in Figure (7). The subject of this book is traditional acupuncture therapy, a use of acupuncture which developed within the context of a system of medicine known as traditional Oriental medicine. Although TOM starts from a different paradigm or conceptual framework than that of Western medicine, both systems share a similar underlying structure, which is in fact the structure of any complete medical system. This structure can be represented by a circle with eight divisions corresponding to the categories enumerated in Figure (8), which I call the Circle.[6] In this chapter I will introduce the eight categories of the Circle, outlining the approach to each one in TCM and LA, and also show how they parallel the categories of Western medicine.

The first category consists of axioms and other basic principles or natural laws underlying TOM. At this level are some assumptions that are

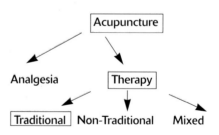

Figure 7:

VARIOUS USES OF ACUPUNCTURE

The most frequent confusion in the popular understanding of acupuncture is due to a failure to distinguish acupuncture analgesia from acupuncture therapy.

quite different from those of contemporary Western medicine, but surprisingly similar to those of its historical antecedents. The first of these

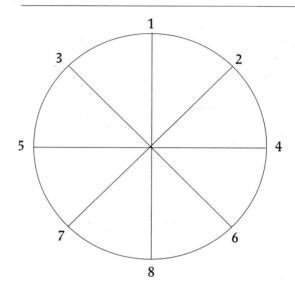

Categories	Western Medicine	TCM	LA
1. Axioms & Laws	Physics & Chemistry	Yin/Yang > 5 Elements Material Substances >Spirit	5 Elements >Yin/Yang Spirit >Material Substances
2. Essential Functions	Physiology	12 Zang Fu Organ Systems	12 Officials
3. Essential Structures	Anatomy	Meridians and Points	Meridians and Points
4. Causes of Illness	Etiology	Exogenous >Endogenous or Miscellaneous Factors	Endogenous >Exogenous or Miscellaneous Factors
5. Nature of Disharmony	Pathology	Qualitative >Quantitative	Quantitative >Qualitative
6. Clinical Investigation	Examination	Four Exams—Overt and Objective	Four Exams—Subjective and Interactive
7. Case Analysis	Diagnosis	Differentiation of Syndromes	Causative Factors
8. Treatment	Therapy	Herbal Orientation	Acupunctural Orientation

Figure 8: THE CIRCLE

This is the model used by the author to compare various styles of medical practice, whether of Western or Eastern origin is the concept of Qi (pronounced "chee"), a Chinese word that merits a different translation for each context in which it is used. Sometimes it means breath, sometimes energy, and often it seems to be synonymous with the vital force or "vis medicatrix naturae" (natural healing force) which was recognized in Western medical circles at least until the nineteenth century. There is a famous Chinese epigram stating that the universe is nothing more nor less than Qi and the laws which govern its behavior. Thus the discussion of basic principles will fall into two subcategories: the fundamental substances, of which Qi is the prototype, and the energetic laws which govern its behavior.[7] TCM places great emphasis on studying the transformations or metabolism of the fundamental substances which are derived from Qi, especially the more tangible ones known as Blood and Fluids (Fig.9). TCM's energetic orientation is primarily the theory of Yin and Yang. LA on the other hand, accepts Qi as the all-inclusive fundamental substance or bodily constituent, but is less interested in the relationships of its derivative forms, singling out for special attention only the least tangible one known as Spirit. LA's energetic orientation is primarily the theory of the Five Elements. If we compare this level of analysis in TOM with its counterpart in Western medicine, we would probably be discussing elementary particles and quantum mechanics as the two corresponding subcategories of natural law. While Western science is currently searching for a unified field theory to encompass the diverse energetic laws it has discovered, TOM has since its inception operated from the intuitively recognized "unified field theories" of Yin/Yang and the Five Elements, though neither of these models can be applied with the mathematical rigor demanded by Western science. There have been a number of books pointing to this similarity of Eastern and Western science, but I think that it is important to maintain a distinction between the two—one synthetic and inductive, the other analytic and deductive. They are complementary ways of perceiving and organizing reality that are not reducible, one to the other.

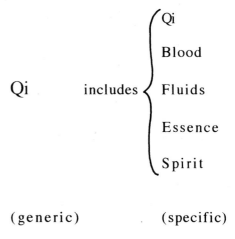

Figure 9: THE BASIC SUBSTANCES
Qi is both the inclusive term for all the vital substances in the body, and also a specific type of bodily substance when used in a more restrictive sense.

The second category of the Circle is the study of the vital functions, of which there are twelve singled out as being of primary importance in TOM. Once again, TCM and LA emphasize different aspects of these twelve. TCM refers to them as "Organs" while LA calls them "Officials." Both approaches however recognize the same twelve traditional components which have names that are already familiar to us such as Lung, Large Intestine, Stomach, etc. These same terms have a fundamentally structural connotation in Western thought, while in TOM it is not their physical make-up, but what they do, that is considered essential, and this priority of function over structure is shared by both TCM and LA.

Every function must be associated, however, with some type of structure, and so the third category of the Circle relates to the human body, starting from those parts associated with the twelve primary functions. Once again, the obvious structural correlations to us Westerners are not the ones of primary concern in TOM. Rather than focussing on the anatomy of the Organs themselves, acupuncturists are most concerned with the regions of the body that each Organ influences. These regions are traversed by invisible but nonetheless meticulously described Meridians or Channels, which among other roles transport the Qi throughout the body (Fig.10). It is also along these Meridian pathways that the acupuncture Points are located, where practitioners insert their needles to alter the flow of Qi, and by this effect are able to influence bodily functions in health and in illness. The objective reality of the Meridians and their Points has never been established to the satisfaction of Western scientists, although there have been numerous suggestive studies.[8] Regardless, these anatomically defined "structures" remain the backbone of the practice of acupuncture. Both TCM and LA emphasize study of the twelve Principal Meridians which are associated with the Organs, whereas several of the less well known styles of acupuncture which I will mention in Chapter Five have focussed on other components of the Meridian system, called "Secondary Vessels," which include the Extraordinary Meridians, the Divergent Meridians, the Connecting Meridians and the Tendinomuscular Meridians.

The fourth category of the Circle is etiology, or the study of the causes of disease. In contrast to Western medicine which posits the basic cause of most disease as being an invasion from without (for example, germs, toxins and allergens) Oriental medicine places more emphasis on the maintainance of health from within. Health is said to be maintained by the activity of Righteous Qi which repels any incursion by pathogenic factors known as Evil Qi. Of course the virulence of pathogenic forces and the strength of host resistance are both important factors to take into account in any system of medicine, but their

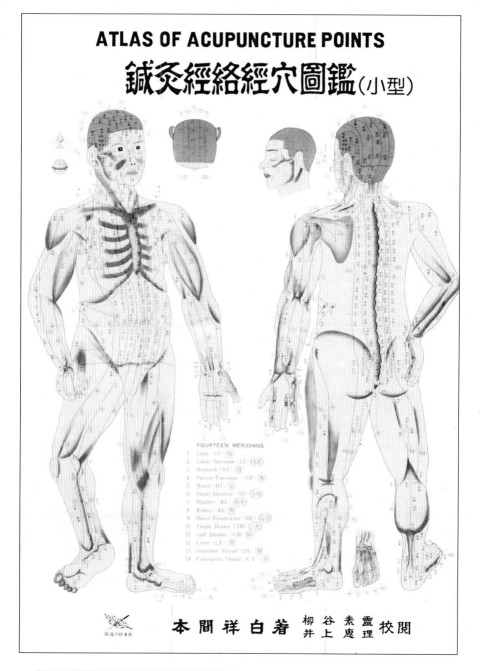

Figure 10: THE ACUPUNCTURE MERIDIANS
Various charts of the Meridians have been drawn by individual authors. This chart by the late Japanese teacher Honma Shohaku artistically illustrates the Points, Meridians and Organs to which they connect internally.

relative primacy varies. The Classics of TOM teach that if a person follows the correct way of life, he will be immune to attacks of illness. A
similar emphasis on the terrain underlying the development of disease
can be found in pre-twentieth century Western medical theory. Having
said this much, it is important to notice that TCM and LA place different emphases on these etiological categories. TCM tends towards a
greater focus on the types of Evil Qi which contest with the Righteous
Qi, for example Wind, Cold or Dampness—whether of Exogenous or
Endogenous origin. LA on the other hand has an almost exclusive interest in the type of malfunction of the Righteous Qi, insofar as it relates
to the Five Elements and their Twelve Officials. The mental, emotional
and spiritual causes for these aberrations are given relatively greater
prominence. This difference in emphasis is in keeping with the general
approaches of TCM as more materialistic and LA as more spiritualistic
in nature.

The fifth category of the Circle is pathology, or the study of the
alterations of the human organism which occur in disease. To some
authors, the development of the science of pathology in the 1800's, as
fathered by Rudolf Virchow, was the crucial factor which allowed for
the emergence of modern Western medicine. I would venture to say
that a parallel development has never occurred in TOM, whose pathological theories remain more elementary. Both TCM and LA recognize
imbalance, per se, as the basic pathological condition, with TCM
focussing more on its qualitative manifestation such as the formation
of abnormal bodily substances including Phlegm and Stagnant Blood,
for example, while LA focussing more on the quantitative imbalances
subsumed under the categories of Excess and Deficiency. These are of
course not absolute differences in approach, but recognizing this distinction is essential to understanding the consequent differences
between the two styles of acupuncture in the realms of examination,
diagnosis and treatment.

Category six involves the methods of examination employed by
acupuncturists, which are traditionally listed as seeing, hearing, questioning and feeling. All of these methods are dependent on the direct
perceptual skills of the practitioner which are therefore the most important part of a practitioner's training. There is very little counterpart to
the use of laboratory and other "third party" methods of examination
and testing which form such an important component of contemporary
Western medicine. Examination is really the process of gathering data,
and in TCM this process is oriented around those preceding issues pertinent to this style: Yin/Yang, the Qi, Blood and Fluids, the Organ functions and the different qualitative types of pathology. The examination
in LA on the other hand, is oriented around the Five Elements, the emo-

tional and spiritual state of the patient, especially with respect to the functions of the twelve Officials, and the quantitative imbalances in the distribution of Qi. This difference is most easily appreciated in the contrasting methods of pulse diagnosis employed by the two styles, to be described in Chapter Two.

From the data gathered by examination, a diagnosis can then be formulated. The hallmark of Western medical diagnosis is naming or identifying the specific disease from which a patient is suffering. In TOM, although this approach to diagnosis does exist, relatively greater emphasis is placed on identifying the energetic mechanism or pattern underlying the specific disease manifestation. Discriminating the pattern in Yin/Yang terms has become formalized in TCM as the "Eight Principles," a short-hand term that is often substituted for TCM much as "Five Elements" is casually used as an interchangeable term for LA. The Eight Principles, or as I prefer to think of them, the Eight Diagnostic Categories will also be spelled out in Chapter Two as will the major diagnostic theory of LA referred to as the Causative Factor.

Finally, based on all the preceding steps, a method of treatment is chosen and carried out. As the subject under discussion is acupuncture, that will be the focus of my presentation, however, I should reiterate that the Chinese word which is usually translated as acupuncture, zhen jiu, actually means the use of needles and cauterization, so a more accurate translation would be acupuncture-moxibustion; but in English that becomes rather unwieldy. Both acupuncture and moxibustion are forms of physical therapy, however the reader should keep in mind that TOM encompasses many other forms of treatment including internal medicines (herbal), diet, meditation and therapeutic exercises to name a few of the more common ones. Other than noting that TCM acupuncture has been strongly influenced by herbal medical practice, with which it is usually conjoined and whose history will therefore also be reviewed, I will not devote much attention to these other methods. In some ways, the differences between TCM and LA style acupuncture can best be appreciated by recognizing this close link between TCM and herbal medicine on one hand, and the absence of any such linkage for LA on the other.

Acupuncture treatment, regardless of the style employed, is aimed at reestablishing balance and harmony to the organism — whether the focus is on Qi and Blood, Yin and Yang, the Five Elements, the Officials, the Organs, the Meridians, or the Body/Mind/Spirit as a whole. It is for that reason that acupuncture is spoken of as a "holistic" modality, in contrast to Western medical treatment which at times can lose sight of the patient as a whole in the process of extirpating his disease. Of course an enlightened and sensitive Western medical practitioner is least likely to commit this type of "error" while there are no shortage of acupuncture practitioners whose own "blind-spots" leave them far short of the goal of holism, so I do not wish to paint a picture in which one type of practice is seen as superior to another—I view them as essentially complementary, and have merely attempted to help the reader understand their differences.

Thus, in summary, the Circle can be seen as encompassing the various steps in the theory and practice of acupuncture. Steps one through five move through the various preclinical disciplines while six through eight carry this movement forward into clinical practice. At each level of the Circle there is a natural correspondence between the left and the right. Thus, we start out at step one with a general philosophy and system of belief which is unitary—both from the perspective of the Dao on which it is based and from the point of view of Qi, the unitary matter-energy which is the practical basis for acupuncture treatment. At step two there are twelve vital functions which correspond to the twelve Principal Meridians of step three. These first three steps can be thought of as describing the condition of the normal human being, free from disease or disorder of any sort. At step four a perturbing force is introduced which produces a corresponding pathological reaction at step five. Thus the equator of the Circle represents the development of an illness. This can either be spontaneously resolved in which case there is a reversion to the top half of the Circle, or the illness may persist untreated in which case we remain at the equator, or finally, medical help may be sought in which case we descend to steps six and seven. Here, an examination is carried out and based on the findings a diagnosis is determined. All the prior steps are now focussed on selecting and carrying out the proper acupuncture treatment at step eight which if successful will restore the perturbed Qi to a state of balance and thereby return the patient to health in the top half of the Circle (Fig.11). This process is predicated on the assumption that when the Qi is in a completely balanced and harmonious state, the organism will heal itself from whatever previous illness it experienced. This is not the place to try to validate acupuncture therapy in a scientific manner, however, there is an enormous body of clinical material supporting such a belief in the efficacy of acupuncture.[9] The implication that any form of pathology is potentially reversible if its energetic basis can be fully determined and if the principles of the regulation of Qi can be understood deeply enough is indeed a challenging one. The next chapter will delve a little deeper into the types of knowledge and skill that allow practitioners of TCM and LA to come closer to this common goal. It will present an overview of how each style, first TCM and then LA approaches each category of the Circle and integrates them in the process of treatment so that the reader will be able to identify which tradition's teachings are being described in the historical analysis which follows. I'd like to mention here my conviction that neither style of acupuncture is better nor more effective than the other, but that each is only as good as the training and skill of its practitioners. Ultimately, both styles evolved from the same source and are best seen as brother and sister rather than as competitors for the truth.

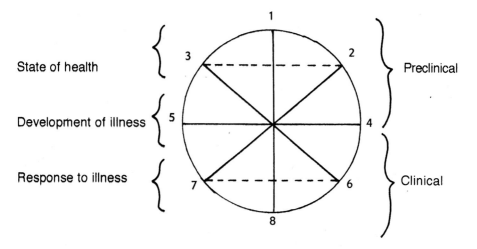

Figure 11: LEVELS OF THE CIRCLE
The model depicted in Figure 8 is expanded to indicate the regions concerned with healthy functioning, the development of "diseases," and the recovery of health through medical intervention.

2

TCM and LA

TCM developed in China under the guiding light of dialectical materialism. As such, it has needed to reject those historical aspects of TOM that reflected spiritual issues, especially practices and attitudes derived from the shamanistic roots of TOM. Essentially it has focussed on somatic complaints and relegated most complaints of mental, emotional and spiritual distress to the realm of politics. Of course there are exceptions to this generalization, but it is a useful distinction in getting a "feel" for TCM.

YIN	YANG
feminine, interior, cold	masculine, exterior, hot
inactive, night, moon	active, day, sun
falling, water, the Earth	rising, fire, Heaven
heavy, dark, damp	light, bright, dry
deficient, front, decreasing	excess, back, increasing
Blood, the Zang, stationary	Qi, the Fu, moving
sedating, material	stimulating, energetic

Figure 12: A COMPARISON OF YIN & YANG
The intuitive appreciation of the differences between the terms in these two columns provides a better understanding of Yin and Yang than would a strict definition.

In keeping with the notion of dialectics, TCM's basic organizing theory is that of Yin and Yang which are themselves a pair of opposites whose mutual attraction, interpentration and self-transformation underlie all developmental processes. The strict meanings of the terms Yin and Yang are surprisingly simple: Yin depicts the shady side and Yang the sunny side of a hill. By implication, all that is cold, dark, wet and inactive exhibits Yin qualities, while all that is hot, bright, dry and active expresses Yang qualities (Fig.12). In a state of health, Yin and Yang ebb and flow harmoniously, and continuously keep each other and themselves in balance. At the level of basic constituents, this bipartite model is used to describe even the Qi itself: Qi is Yang with respect to Blood, but at the same time Qi is Yin with respect to Spirit. Thus, it's essential to keep in mind that Yin and Yang are relative terms and one must always know the context in order to understand their specific meanings. Figure (13) shows the relationships of the five basic bodily constituents and how they are related to each other in Yin/Yang terms.

In its strictest sense, Qi is a specific one of the five basic constituents, while in a broader sense Qi can also be used to refer to all five at once. Thus, not only Yin and Yang, but even Qi changes its meaning depending on context. This close connection between the concepts of Qi, Yin and Yang is illustrated by the similarity in ancient Chinese characters for these three terms (Fig.14)[10].

The materialistic approach of TCM which operates from category one of the Circle, is immediately felt at category two, where the twelve basic functions are expressed as Solid and Hollow Organs[11]. Thus these twelve Organs are understood in terms of their relationships to the basic bodily constituents. For example, the Lungs rule the Qi and adjust the Fluid Channels while the Liver stores the Blood and smooths the flow of Qi. Because the Organs have these physical roles to play, illnesses are frequently seen as being manifestations of disorder in carrying out these functions. At the level of category three, the acupuncture Points are often classified in terms of their effects on the basic constituents, such as Points for regulating the Blood and other Points for tonifying the Qi. In category four, the main etiological factors are the six climatic excesses: Wind, Cold, Damp, Dryness, Heat and Fire. While it is acknowledged that emotional upsets can be a cause of illness, there is no systematic application of this knowledge to how emotions affect the categories on other levels of the Circle, information that by comparison is well articulated for the climatic excesses. As mentioned, physical pathologies such as Phlegm or Stagnant Blood are often specified as explanations of the disease mechanism in category five and are seen as resulting partly from retention and transformation of one or more of the preceding six factors. These etiologic and pathologic factors can be identified by the observant practitioner during the examination which is category six. For example, Stagnant Blood manifests as purple discoloration on the surface of the body, particularly on the tongue, and is characterized by severe stabbing pains, worse from pressure and aggravated at night, and presents a

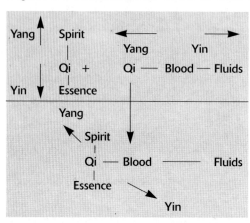

Figure 13: YIN & YANG OF THE BASIC SUBSTANCES
The five Basic Substances participate in two trinities: a homeostatic metabolic process governed by Qi, Blood and Fluids, and an evolutionary developmental process governed by Essence, Qi and Spirit. Each can be described in Yin/Yang terms.

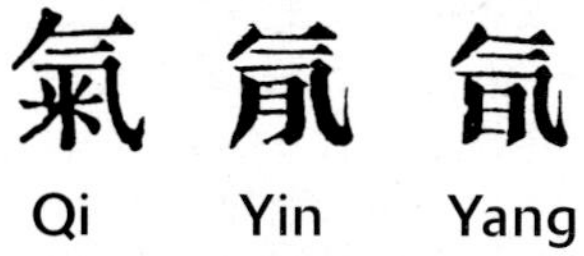

氣 氚 氤

Qi   Yin   Yang

Figure 14: ANCIENT CHINESE CHARACTERS

for Qi, Yin & Yang share 气 which indicates some kind of vapor or unseen force, and which has become the modern Chinese character for Qi itself. Where Yin and Yang have symbols for the moon and sun respectively, Qi has the symbol for rice, the physical basis for energy. *(See Faubert, page 22)* pulse which is hesitant or choppy in quality (Fig.15). Thus one of the tasks of diagnosis, in category seven, is to determine by examination which of the various etiological and/or pathological factors are present. Such a determination is made by looking for a typical pattern, as for example the pattern of Stagnant Blood just described. This type of pattern discrimination is not used just to identify the etiologic and pathologic factors, but also to determine the location and other attributes of the disease process. The most common diagnostic rubric employed in TCM is referred to as the Eight Principles, which is shorthand for the Eight Principles for Discriminating Patterns[12], and it is this attempt to discriminate patterns which is characteristic of all diagnoses in TOM. The Eight Principles are: Hot, Cold, Excess, Deficient, Exterior, Interior, Yin and Yang. It is clear that a diagnosis restricted to these eight patterns alone would however be incomplete, as we need to know which aspect of the organism is being affected. Thus, in addition to discriminating which of the eight patterns are present, the diagnosis also needs to discriminate which Organs or Meridians are involved. For example a simple, yet complete TCM diagnosis in a patient presenting with chronic diarrhea, abdominal bloating, pale tongue and an empty pulse might be Deficiency of Qi of the Spleen—which is an Interior, Deficient, Cold and Yin pattern (Fig.16). This amount of diagnostic specificity allows for the selection of an appropriate acupuncture treatment prescription in category eight of the Circle. A typical protocol for the

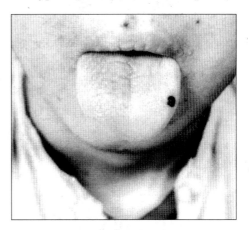

Figure 15: STAGNANT BLOOD.
This patient's tongue shows a prominent ecchymotic spot on the edge which is indicative of Blood stagnation.

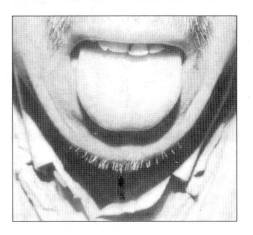

Figure 16:
DEFICIENCY OF QI OF THE SPLEEN.
The typical appearance of the tongue in this condition is shown: a pale tongue body with a thin white coat.

pattern just described might be to insert needles at the following acupuncture Points: Stomach 36, Spleen 3, Conception Vessel 12 and Bladder 20 (Fig.17). The needles would be manipulated with tonifying technique[13] and left in place for about 20 minutes. This or a similar protocol might be repeated frequently over the course of a few weeks, after which it would be

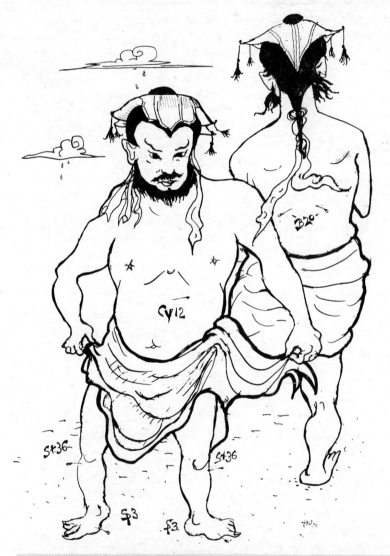

Figure 17: Treatment for Deficient Spleen Qi
There is no single "correct" treatment, but rather a range of possibilities for each condition, and the practitioner must choose the best one for the individual patient. This illustration shows a seven needle treatment that promotes balance between left and right, front and back, upper and lower and Yin and Yang Meridians, while tonifying the Qi of the Spleen.

expected that the diarrhea would have stopped and the tongue and pulse findings would have shifted in the direction of normality. Should this not be the case, it would be grounds for reevaluating the initial examination and diagnosis. When the symptoms have resolved, and the pulse and tongue findings are more normal, the patient would be considered "cured" and be given specific advice as to lifestyle—in this case diet in particular— so as to avoid a recurrence.

By contrast, LA, incorporating material from all over the Orient as well as from the West, was systematized in England with an emphasis on just those aspects of TOM which were rejected by TCM in China. Of central importance in this regard is the role of Spirit, which is seen as the true captain of the assemblage making up a human being: Body, Mind and Spirit. Many passages from the classics of TOM attest to this primacy, e.g.,

> "The Yellow Emperor asked Qi Bo saying, "The laws of acupuncture dictate that needling should be, first and foremost, based upon the Spirit .. . . ."[14]

Just what is implied by the term Spirit can however, only be hinted at, but never fully articulated. In another passage,

> "Qi Bo answered: Let me explain the Spirit. What is the Spirit? The Spirit cannot be heard with the ear. The eye must be brilliant of perception and the Heart must be open and attentive, and then the Spirit is suddenly revealed through one's own consciousness. It cannot be expressed through the mouth; only the Heart can express all that can be looked upon. If one pays close attention, one may suddenly know it but one can just as suddenly lose this knowledge. But the Spirit becomes clear to man as though the wind has blown away the cloud"[15].

Many aspects of LA reflect this emphasis on the Spirit. These include everything from enumerating specific acupuncture Points which have a special power to affect the Spirit, to a coordinated acupuncture protocol for exorcizing cases of spiritual "possession." As we shall see, historically demonology and exorcism have traditionally been a part of acupuncture, probably reflecting the practitioners' early forebears who were the shamen in ancient China. Closely tied to its emphasis on Spirit is a recognition of the importance of the mind and emotions in health and illness. These are incorporated in LA as part of the Five Element theory which I am about to discuss, but I want to point out first that this attention to thoughts and feelings, that is, the inner life of human beings, is probably the greatest attraction of LA for Westerners. Of course it is understandable that such a focus on the subtleties of each individual's intellectual and emotional life might seem to be incompatible with the political situation in China, and could easily account for its absence from TCM. The Five Element theory provides an excellent organizing tool, going back to category one, for LA's focus on the Spirit, Mind and Emotions. Five Element theory is a bit more complex than Yin/Yang theory, so I'll present a few more details of it application. Like Yin and Yang, the Five Elements[16] can in the first place be thought of as a mechanism for classifying all phenomena into separate categories, each of which share some kind of mutual resonance, much as do cold, dark and wet in the classification called Yin (Fig.18). The Five Elements are Wood, Fire, Earth, Metal and Water. So, for example, Wind, Spring, the Liver, green, sour and rancid are all associated by resonance with the element Wood. There are various sequences in which the Elements occur with respect to different phenomena relating to acupuncture. The most common sequence, which I have given, is called the Creative cycle and repeats itself endlessly (Fig.19). Because in category two, the Twelve Organs are correlated to the Five Elements, this Creative cycle is invoked to explain how the Liver, for example, supports and nourishes the Heart, which in turn nourishes the Spleen (Fig.20), etc.

There is also a Control cycle in which the Elements and their associated Organs inhibit or restrain each other as in Figure 21.

	WOOD	FIRE	EARTH	METAL	WATER
DIRECTION	East	South	Center	West	North
CLIMATE	Wind	Heat	Damp	Dry	Cold
FLAVOR	Sour	Bitter	Sweet	Pungent	Salty
ZANG	Liver	Heart Pericardium	Spleen	Lungs	Kidneys
FU	GallBladder	Three Heater Small Intestine	Stomach	Large Intestine	Bladder
TISSUE	Tendons	Vessels	Flesh	Skin	Bones
SENSE ORGAN	Eyes	Tongue	Mouth	Nose	Ears
EMOTION	Anger	Joy	Sympathy	Grief	Fear
ODOR	Rancid	Scorched	Fragrant	Rotten	Putrid
SOUND	Shouting	Laughing	Singing	Weeping	Groaning
COLOR	Green	Red	Yellow	White	Blue
SEASON	Spring	Summer	Indian Summer	Autumn	Winter
STAGE	Birth	Growth	Transformation	Decline	Storage

Figure 18: CORRELATES OF THE FIVE ELEMENTS.

Not all compilations of the Five Element associations are in agreement, this list reflecting the associations that are made in LA. The most controversial entries are the colors for Wood (often stated to be Blue-Green) and Water (often stated to be Black) and the emotion for Earth (often stated to be pensiveness).

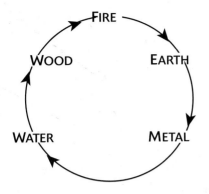

Of course whole books can be written on Five Element theory, but for present purposes, I just want to introduce enough information from its core concepts, since it is the basic organizing theory of LA in category one, to allow the reader to appreciate the history which follows. At category two I have been referring to the Organs, but I ought here to call them the Officials, which is the term used

Figure 19: THE CREATIVE CYCLE OF THE FIVE ELEMENTS
This cycle flows clockwise (the apparent direction of the sun through the Heavens) and illustrates how each Element engenders the succeeding Element, much as a parent creates (and nourishes) a child. Thus, an alternate name for the relationships depicted in this cycle is the "Law of Mother-Son."

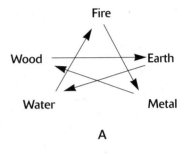

A

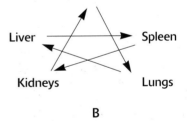

B

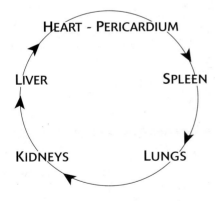

Figure 20: THE CREATIVE CYCLE OF THE ZANG ORGANS
In the language of the Law of Mother-Son, for example, the Lungs are the Mother of the Kidneys and the Son of the Spleen, while the Kidneys are the Son of the Lungs and the Mother of the Liver.

Figure 21: THE CONTROL CYCLE OF THE FIVE ELEMENTS (A) & THE ZANG ORGANS (B)
Each Element or Organ controls the one located two positions further along in a clockwise direction, and is in turn controlled by the one located two positions prior in a counter-clockwise direction. For example, Fire controls Metal, but is controlled by Water; the Liver controls the Spleen, but is controlled by the Lungs.

in LA. It is derived from Chapter Eight of the *Su Wen* which compares the functions of the human organism to the administration of a state. Thus, the twelve Officials are:

I	Heart - Supreme Controller
II	Small Intestine - Transformer of Matter and Separator of the Pure from the Impure
III	Bladder - Controller of the Storage of Water
IV	Kidney - Controller of Water
V	Circulation/Sex (Pericardium) - Protector of the Heart
VI	Three Heater - Official of Balance and Harmony
VII	Gallbladder - Decision-Maker and Judge
VIII	Liver - Controller of Planning
IX	Lung - Receiver of the Pure Qi of Heaven
X	Colon - Drainer of the Dregs
XI	Stomach - Controller of Rottening and Ripening
XII	Spleen - Controller of Transport

Figure 22: THE TWELVE OFFICIALS
as administrators of the human "state."

The Officials, being personifications of the twelve functions, are more easily related to in terms of Body, Mind and Spirit than mere Organs would be. At the level of structure, category three, even the acupuncture Points partake of this personification. The traditional Point names, which are quite ancient, are seen as embodying the Spirits of the individual Points. Thus the Point Liver 14, Gate of Hope, might be an important site for treatment in a case of depression and despair, particularly if suggested by other confirmatory diagnostic findings. For this reason, in LA it is important to learn the names of all 361 Points as was traditionally done, rather than just their modern alphanumerical classification. As for etiology, category four, instead of focussing on the six climatic factors which are classified as exogenous Evils, LA is mostly concerned with the so-called seven emotional factors which are traditionally classified as the endogenous Evils. There are various versions of the seven emotions, but LA concentrates on five specific emotions which have a fixed association with the Five Elements. Thus Wood is associated with anger, Fire with joy, Earth with sympathy, Metal with grief and Water with fear. The concept is that any emotion when expressed or suppressed beyond the normal healthy range might then become a source of illness. LA teaches that in the modern world, where most individuals have at least adequate food, shelter and clothing, our persistent susceptibility to both acute and chronic illnesses is more a reflection of the emotional damages transmitted through our Minds and Spirits, than through any Evil factors attacking our Bodies. The resulting pathologies are usually inhibition (Deficiency) or overexcitation (Excess) of any of the twelve Officials in the majority of cases, while more serious pathology might involve various forms of energetic pollution such as "Aggressive Energy," "Demonic Possession" or "Husband-Wife" imbalances. These latter three pathological entities are not included in the lexicon of TCM, and the whole concept of pollution is again more reminiscent of a shamanistic heritage where purification rites were an important part of the ritual of healing. The examination, category six, in LA is naturally organized around the Five Elements. Its most important aspects include determining the presence or absence of subtle colors, odors, vocal qualities and emotional tendencies which correlate with the Five Elements as in Figure 18.

As in TCM, the examination of the pulse is of major importance in LA, but rather than focussing on the various pulse qualities, the important point is now the overall strength or weakness of the radial pulse at the different positions correlated to the twelve Officials. LA does not emphasize examination of the tongue, but instead employs various techniques such as abdominal palpation and Akabane testing[17] of the Meridians which are not commonly used in TCM. By using its own methods of examination, LA gathers the necessary information to make a diagnosis, which almost always includes a determination of which Element and/or Official has been most seriously imbalanced, which now becomes designated as the Causative Factor, or CF. Other ancillary diagnostic findings may include the level of Body, Mind or Spirit at which the imbalance is manifest, and the presence of any of the special cases of pollution (or other special situations which are included in the category called blocks in LA) mentioned above. As an example, the hypothetical patient whose case was presented in the description of TCM involving abdominal bloating and diarrhea might also be likely to have a yellowish complexion, singing voice, fragrant odor and craving for attention and sympathy. Of course all these signs need not be present, but if this pattern seems evident, then the patient would be diagnosed as having an Earth Causative Factor. Careful questioning into the vicissitudes of his private life might reveal a particularly devastating disappointment by his mother at a formative age with an unwillingness to fully engage himself in life from that time onwards. Diagnostically, this could indicate an imbalance of the Earth Element at the Spirit level, and while the treatment protocol used in TCM might be effective in stopping the diarrhea, the case would not be considered successfully treated in LA unless the Spirit was restored as well. This might occur in the course of routine treatment, which in LA involves transferring energy into the Deficient Earth Officials from those Officials found to have Excess Qi, or a hyperfunctional state of excitation on the pulse. In order to transfer energy, use is made of the Creative and Control cycles of the Five Elements and their association with the Five Element or Command Points on each Meridian.[18] For instance, if the Heart and Small Intestine

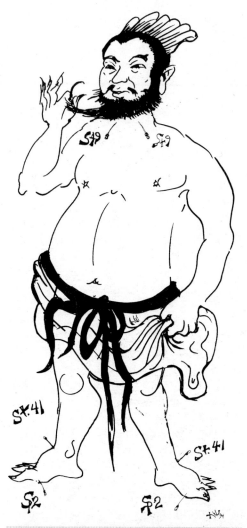

Figure 23: TREATMENT FOR AN EARTH CAUSATIVE FACTOR

In LA as in TCM there is no single "correct" treatment for each diagnosis, but a range of possibilities that must be considered for the individual patient. This illustration shows a six needle treatment in which the Points on the feet help transfer energy from the Fire to the Earth Element, while the Point on the neck focusses this extra energy to assist in the recovery of the patient's Spirit.

had Excess energy, then a typical treatment would involve tonifying the Fire points of the Earth Officials, i.e. Points Spleen 2 and Stomach 41. Needles are typically removed immediately following stimulation in this method. Only if this routine approach to energetic balancing failed to accomplish the goals of treatment after a reasonable period of time would a special Point with more potent access to the Spirit such as a "Window of the Sky Point," Stomach 9 for example, be employed (Fig.23). Each treatment would be monitored for immediate changes in color, sound, odor, emotion and pulses indicating an improved state of balance. Treatment might be continued intermittently over a longer period of time once the presenting symptoms were under control until the underlying spiritual injury began to heal. Only then would the case be considered successfully treated, and the patient might be advised to return for evaluation periodically at the changing of the seasons, for instance, to correct any minor energetic imbalances that might occur.

3

Legendary Lessons in Virtue

In the Orient a legend, fairy tale or myth might begin with the phrase "Back in the time when tigers used to smoke," which would be roughly equivalent to our "once upon a time" (Fig.24). We can think of "smoking tiger time" in two different ways: either as "long, long ago," or alternatively, as something like the aboriginal "dream-time" which is always right now in an alternate view of reality. It is this latter interpretation which I would like to emphasize in beginning this history book with what might be called a folk-tale.

Like other cultures, the Chinese have a creation myth: before the beginning, there was nothing but chaos, existing in a timeless state and stateless time. Then slowly, chaos began to solidify itself into a colossal stone, within which formed a cosmic egg, and the egg gave birth to a creature, named Pangu (Fig.25). For 18,000 years, Pangu labored to separate the two parts of stone which gave him birth, and these he pushed apart, growing at the rate of ten feet a day. One of these parts became Heaven and the other became Earth, with Pangu himself

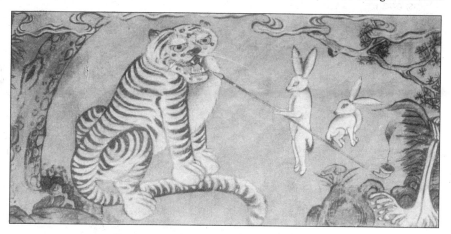

Figure 24: THE SMOKING TIGER,
a Korean folk theme in which the wily rabbit tricks the powerful tiger
(perhaps by inducing an altered state of reality?)

becoming the pillar between them. Eventually he died, and his two eyes became the sun and moon, his breath the wind and clouds, his voice the thunder, his body and limbs the mountains, his bones the stones and minerals, his flesh the soil, his blood the rivers and seas, his hair the trees and flowers, and his fleas and lice the ancestors of all living creatures, including you and me[19].

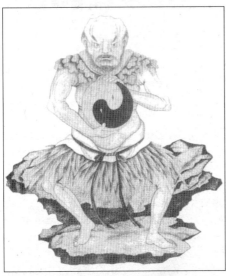

Figure 25: PANGU,
the primordial being who evolved from chaos, and in turn was transformed into the entirety of creation. He is holding the Yin/Yang symbol which represents the force that brings order out of chaos.

The Daoist philosopher Zhuang Zi relates another version of the demise of Chaos, who is identified as Hun-tun, the Emperor of the Center[20]: The Emperor of the South was called Shu, the Emperor of the North was called Hu, and the Emperor of the Center was called Hun-tun[21]. Shu and Hu at times mutually came together and met in Hun-tun's territory. Hun-tun treated them very generously. Shu and Hu, then, discussed how they could reciprocate Hun-tun's virtue, saying: "Men all have seven openings in order to see, hear, eat and breathe. He alone doesn't have any. Let's try boring him some." Each day they bored one hole, and on the seventh day Hun-tun died.

For a long time I have been fascinated by Zhuang Zi's version of this tale without knowing quite what it meant. In the prologue to one of his books, Stan Steiner gives an interpretation that seems to both explain the tale's meaning and also indicate the spirit in which I have tried to approach writing about historical matters:

> "No one can say what another human should be. If one human being tries to make other human beings into his own image, he shall surely kill them. This is true even of gods. And it is true of people in a book, who are made of paper and words. Maybe more so. When a writer describes people and tells their story, if that writer recreates them in his or her own image, the story may be successful but the people may not survive, except as shadows of the writer's ego."[22]

With that in mind, let me point out that there is a very fuzzy line between the realms of mythology, legend and history. This book is primarily about history, but history's own origin lies in the nebulous world of myth. Myths captivate us partly because they deal with the symbolic and poetic, which have a timeless character, allowing even old myths to seem quite contemporary. Thus, the story of poor Hun-tun was given a modern twist in this poem by the Zen monk Han Shan (Fig.26):

> How pleasant were our bodies
> in the days of Chaos
> Needing neither to eat or piss!
> Who came along with his drill,
> And bored us full of these nine
> holes?[23]
> Morning after morning we
> must dress and eat
> Year after year, fret over taxes,
> A thousand of us scrambling
> for a penny,
> We knock our heads together
> and yell for dear life.[24]

Back in 1984 I was asked to give a brief presentation to the annual conference of the Traditional Acupuncture Foundation in Columbia, Maryland. Shortly before coming to Maryland, while I was supposed to be preparing my speech, I came down with the flu. The most I could manage to do was to lie in bed and read, and the book I had in hand at the time was *The Chinese Heritage* by K.C. Wu. It covered a period of about 2500 years, and told the story of the kings who ruled China starting in antiquity. You know how it is when you're feverish—all I could think

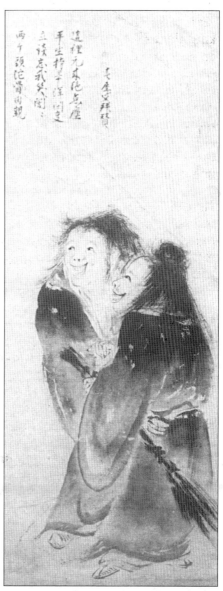

FIGURE 26: HAN SHAN & SHI-DE, Zen (Chan) monks of the Tang dynasty whose irreverence for social mores harkened back to the Daoist ideal of spontaneous simplicity or chaos. They are commonly portrayed as lunatics.

about was those 25 centuries of ancient Chinese kings, so when I got to Maryland, that's what I talked about.

Now, I only had about a half-hour to speak, so for 25 hundred years of kings, that worked out to about 83 years per minute and a new king about every ten seconds. . . .You may think I'm only joking, but I do have a serious point to make, which is that traditional thought in China was fundamentally different from our modern Western way of thinking, and this distinction applies even to the concept of time. Time was not something that could be understood by being measured, but rather by seeing how different times have their own distinctive natures, just as different places do. Thus, the nature or quality of some period of time—be it a king's reign or the length of a dynasty—was much more important than how many years, decades or even centuries were involved. A year could equal a century if their natures were the same. Thus, time was a relative issue, bringing into coordination the time-scale of the universe with that of man. The universe was spoken of as the Macrocosm, while man was felt to be a parallel Microcosm. The two realms obeyed the same fundamental laws or principles, and this was true for notions of both time and space.

Where did these traditional ideas come from? We don't really know, because their origin goes back before the invention of writing— before recorded history. Can you imagine living in a time without written records? "Record" comes from the Latin recordari, to call to mind, which is itself composed of two roots: "re," again and "cor," heart. Thus, Latin tells us that the mind is associated with the activity of the heart over time, and this is virtually the same concept as that of the ancient Chinese who used the same word, xin, (心) for both heart and mind, and considered it the "king" of all the components of the human microcosm.

Another way of communicating ideas is through pictures, as illustrated in the the word heart above, which actually formed the basis for Chinese writing, as opposed to our Western languages, which are alphabetic rather than pictorial. I'll be using a lot of illustrations, partly to make up for this linguistic imbalance. The most well-known pictures in the field of acupuncture are, of course, the charts of the Meridians, as in Figure (27). This shows a contemporary Chinese illustration of what is called the Bladder Meridian, the pathway connecting the acupuncture Points on the surface of the body which the ancient Chinese described as having a relationship to the Urinary Bladder. Of course, the ancient Meridian charts looked somewhat different (Fig.28). I much prefer looking at the latter, but I'm rather old-fashioned. I've often wondered at this gentleman's distinctive headdress. Images which come to mind are a rooster's comb and the heat-dissipat-

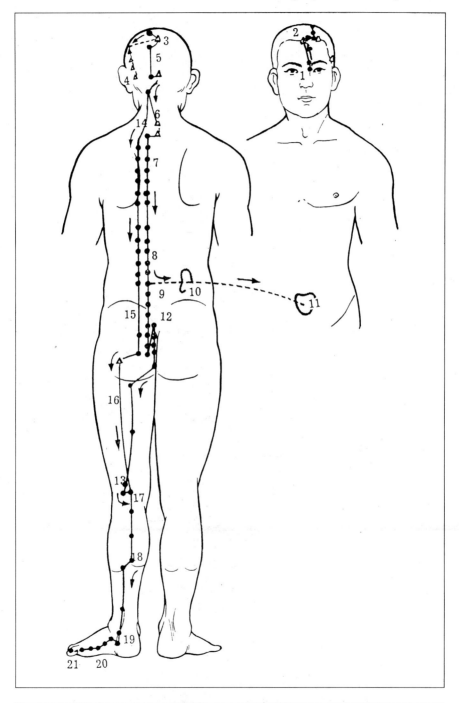

Figure 27: THE BLADDER MERIDIAN.
A contemporary rendition that emphasizes anatomical relationships.

ing fins of the stegosaurus. In a moment of feverish delirium, I even saw him as a "punk mandarin," no disrespect intended. Actually, I've seen quite a few similar looking characters on the streets of London and San Francisco lately (Fig.29)—it's the "Mohawk" look, which brings to mind an old theory, that the American Indians and the Chinese share a common origin—back in this period before recorded history. Wouldn't it be something if it turned out that Americans originally discovered acupuncture? Although I've yet to identify the mysterious headgear, I

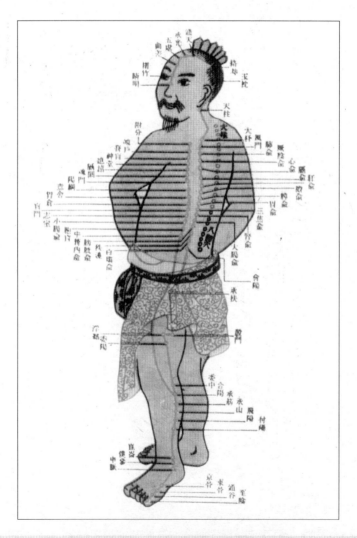

Figure 28: THE BLADDER MERIDIAN.
A more traditional rendition that emphasizes the poetic names of each of the acupuncture Points which lie on its path.

did come across the following brilliant hypothesis in a widely-read American journal (Fig.30).

Now I've shown you that history can be fun, but it has its serious side, too. I chose the topic of the Chinese Kings because it illustrates the role of virtue in traditional Chinese thought. In the West, we're used to separating morality, which falls in the field of religion, from the disciplines of sociology and medicine which we think of as sciences. Traditional Chinese thought did not make this distinction— nothing was profane, every act was sacred. This idea was

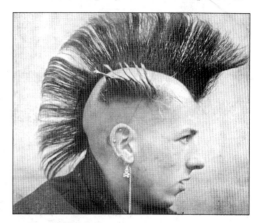

Figure 29: THE "MOHAWK" LOOK, one of the more extreme examples of "New Wave" fashion which emerged among the youth counter-culture in the 1980's.

embodied in the concept of the Three Powers: Heaven was the source of virtue, which in acting on Earth, produced Man and all the 10,000 beings as a consequence. Man was thus the central factor in the cosmos, and depending on how he behaved, so would go the world. I think in our hearts we all know this is true, and yet how far we are from acting on it. Anyway, for the Chinese, the representative of Man, as the central factor, was the King, who was called the Son of Heaven. If his virtue was pure, Heaven gave him its mandate to rule, but if he ceased to be virtuous, Heaven would just as easily remove the mandate and pass it on to another.

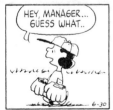 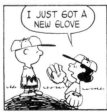 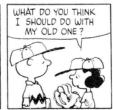 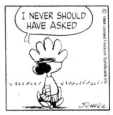

Peanuts reprinted by permission of UFS, Inc.

Figure 30: MANDARINS AND MOHAWKS
Charlie Brown supplies a possible connecting link in this strip by one of America's favorite cartoonists.

This idea of the crucial role of virtue was not confined to politics and history. For example, Chapters 13 and 14 of the oldest and most revered text on Chinese medicine the *Su Wen*, include the following discussion between the Yellow Emperor, Huang Di, and his esteemed teacher Qi Bo:

> "Huang Di said: In ancient times, diseases were cured by prayers alone . . . , but nowadays, physicians treat disease with herbs . . . and acupuncture . . . and the disease is sometimes cured and sometimes not cured. Why? Qi Bo answered: the ancient people lived. . . with neither internal burden of wishes and envies nor external burden of chasing after fame and profit, it was a life of tranquility which made them immune from the deep intrusion of vicious energies... Nowadays. . . they worry a great deal, they work too hard, they fail to follow the climates. . . they have lowered their moral standards, with the result that they are under the attack of vicious energies frequently. . . and when the patient's spirits are not positive, and when their will and sentiments are not stable, the disease cannot recover."

Thus, whether talking about a person or a state, the principles are the same. Sick nations are just like sick patients in this regard, and need to embrace virtue, if they are to prosper. Keep in mind this close parallel between medicine and history and its emphasis on virtue as I begin my story in the distant past, before written records were kept.

Figure (31) shows an overview of 5,000 years of Chinese history, from legendary times all the way to the present century. I've indicated the successive dynasties and their dates, along with some outstanding individuals and their accomplishments. The present chapter introduces the first half of this period, when the mode of thought characteristic of traditional China was being crystallized. Several important figures, Fu Xi and Shen Nong, belonging to the early legendary phase of Chinese history will be discussed in Chapter Four, but the story of the Kings more properly begins with the later Yellow Emperor, Huang Di, who is credited with the discovery of both acupuncture and writing (Fig.32). In fact, Huang Di is the dividing line between China's epoch of legendary Culture Heroes and its actual recorded history, which starts with a series of Premier Emperors and Sage Kings.[25]

The early historical record was pieced together by China's outstanding historians among whom were Confucius and Si Ma Qian. They are both good examples of how seriously the traditional Chinese valued their concept of virtue. From the time of the Yellow Emperor there were officials called "shi" or scribes who always accompanied the ruler. One stayed on his left side, and wrote down everything the ruler said. The other stayed to the right, and wrote down everything the ruler

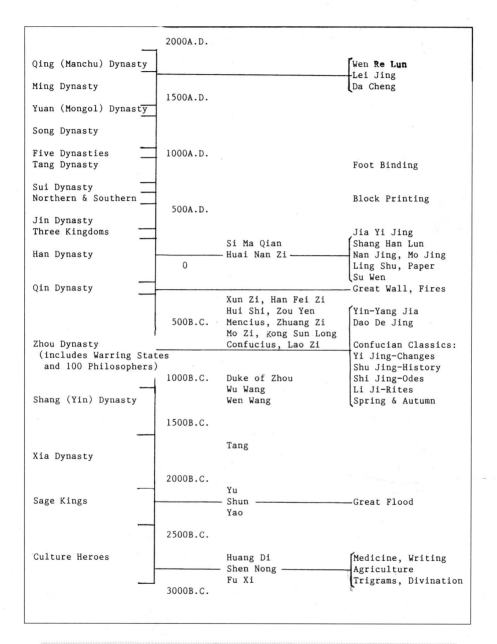

Figure 31: AN OVERVIEW OF CHINESE HISTORY.
This chart presents a highly condensed glimpse of Chinese history from its inception through the fall of its last dynasty, the Qing in 1911.

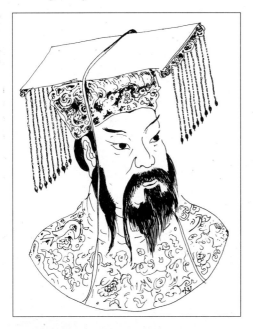

Figure 32: HUANG DI, THE YELLOW EMPEROR.

Yellow is the color associated with the middle, and China is referred to as the "Middle Kingdom" (Zhong Guo), so the Yellow Emperor is symbolically the founder of the Chinese nation. He is legendarily credited with originating acupuncture.

did. Naturally, this could get a scribe in trouble if the Emperor did something he'd rather not have known. Several times scribes were reported to have recorded how their lords murdered their predecessors and were themselves killed for their honesty. It was a rule that scribes should never record anything unless they were absolutely sure of the facts. Indeed, Confucius remarked that when he was young, he was still able to see a scribe leave a blank in his text, meaning the material to be recorded could not be verified. This absolute fidelity was the model, but was dying out even by Confucius' time. Si Ma Qian (Fig.33), a later historian (c. 145–85 B.C.) was himself descended from several generations of scribes, and would not take even Confucius' word as authoritative. He visited every place Confucius had mentioned and rechecked the tablet records in the dynastic archives dating back to the Yellow Emperor, before writing his *Historical Records*. In the end, he fell into disfavor with the Emperor for writing something unflattering, and himself suffered castration and imprisonment rather than repudiate his word.[26]

This office of scribe, record-keeper or librarian-shi was supposedly occupied in his day by Lao Zi, the founder of Daoism and author of *The Way and its Virtue*[27] In his official capacity, Lao Zi was reputed to have met and instructed Confucius, who had come to study the official archives (Fig.34).

The next period of history after Huang Di, famous for its lessons on virtue, is that of the Sage Kings: Yao, Shun and Yu. This was the period of the great flood, probably the same as that described in the Bible, which was threatening to destroy the world around 2300 B.C. Every year the flooding got worse—it just kept raining, and there was nowhere for the water to go. Yao was the Emperor, and he came to the realization that he could not stop the floods—the situation was beyond him (Fig.35). He decided to give China (which to him was the world) to anyone who could control the floods. The man he found was Shun, whose only claim to fame was his perfect virtue (Fig.36). He exemplified the cardinal virtue, to the Chinese, of filial piety. Frankly, Shun came from an absolutely awful family. His parents and siblings made him do all the work and then heaped

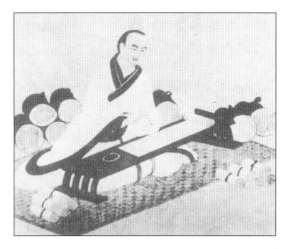

Figure 33: SI MA QIAN, THE GRAND HISTORIAN. He was a meticulous scribe who based his writings on both literary research and firsthand interviews, and we owe much of our knowledge of early Chinese history to his endeavours.

abuse on him, and when he didn't complain, that really enraged them, and they decided to kill him. They sent him up to work on the roof of the barn, and then they set fire to it. Miraculously, Shun escaped by using a pair of large bamboo hats as parachutes to break his fall when

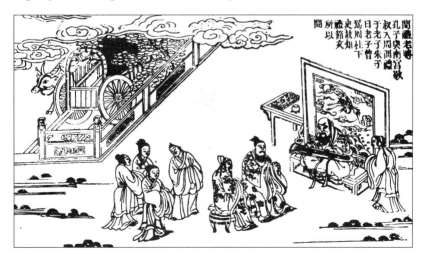

Figure 34: LAO ZI AND CONFUCIUS.
Daoist legend claims that Confucius consulted Lao Zi on a question of ritual while the latter was an archival official.

he jumped. Did that get Shun mad? No. Next, his family set him to dig a well, and when he was digging below ground, they covered him up—just buried him alive! Of course, by now Shun was on to their tricks and had already dug an escape tunnel in advance, so he foiled them again, and all this without ever creating any trouble himself.

So, Emperor Yao figured if anyone could save China it might be Shun, because of his perfect virtue—mind you, not because he knew the least thing about flood control! Yao offered the Empire to Shun and Shun refused it—he didn't think himself worthy. Finally, he allowed himself to be persuaded to become co-emperor with Yao. Together they searched for the best engineer, who turned out to be Yu, the founder of the Xia dynasty (Fig.37). Yu directed the dredging of the great rivers to deepen them. By "moving mountains" and "changing the course of rivers," Yu saved the country. Yu's virtue centered not on filial piety, but on goodness or compassion, meaning a sense of responsibility for the sufferings of others, to the point of simply not being able to bear that others should suffer. It was said of Yu, that if anyone drowned as a result of the flood, he felt as if it were he himself that had drowned him. Yu's labors on flood control lasted thirteen years, during which time he was so pressed with work that he never once was able to visit his home and family, including his infant son who would become heir to the Xia dynasty.[29] The story of Yu's virtue is one that I think is most pertinent for those in the healing professions to ponder.[30]

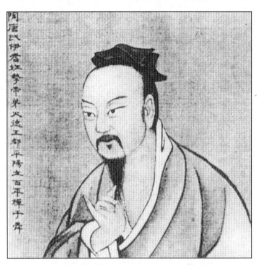

Figure 35: EMPEROR YAO,
the first of the Sage Kings in the time of the great flood. His story begins the *Classic of History (Shu Jing)*.

The Xia dynasty was succeeded by the Shang or Yin dynasty, which flourished until around 1100 B.C. It was ushered in around 1800 B.C. by King Tang, also famous for his virtue, but by 1100 B.C. the dynastic virtue had deteriorated to where an absolute demon, Zou, was on the throne. Here was a man who disemboweled pregnant women to satisfy his curiosity as to the sex of their offspring! I can't even bring myself to

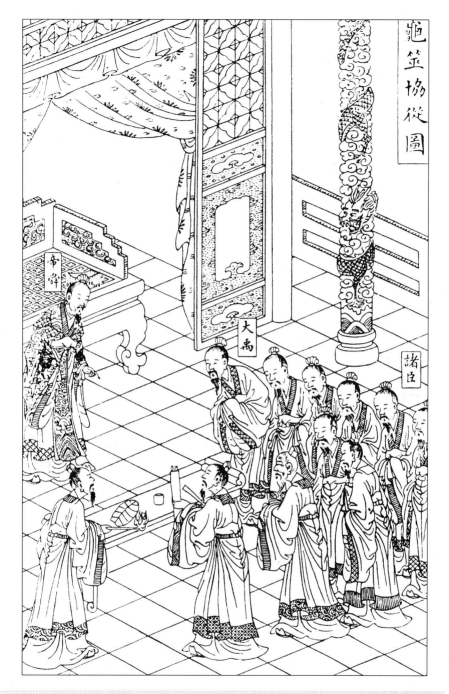

Figure 36: EMPEROR SHUN, THE EXEMPLAR OF FILIAL PIETY.
He is shown with his ministers (including Yu) conducting a divination in which a heated rod will be applied to a tortoise shell to produce a pattern of significant cracks.

See Figure 41 and the accompanying text for a more complete description of this ceremony.

relate any of the other atrocities that he committed—it was time for Heaven to remove the mandate.

There was, at this time, a scholarly noble, King Wen of Zhou, who was trying to administer his domain in a virtuous manner. Naturally, the wicked king Zou saw him as a threat, and had him thrown in jail for several years. But this was a man who did not waste time. He took his imprisonment as an opportunity to meditate, and then wrote the 64 hexagrams and their commentaries which form the *Yi Jing* or *Book of Changes*.[31] Zou foolishly took this as a sign of weakness and released him, but Wen Wang's son Wu Wang, the Martial Emperor, overthrew Zou and established the Zhou dynasty. Wen Wang's fourth son, the Duke of Zhou, was his collaborator in writing the *Yi Jing*, and the author of much of the material that eventually became part of the Confucian classics. The Zhou dynasty continued through the time of Confucius and Lao Zi until it, in turn, fell to the Qin dynasty.

What I've presented in this chapter is a brief glimpse at the legacy of Huang Di, the Yellow Emperor, from the dawn of history proper (around 2700 B.C.) down the ages through the eras of the Sage Kings and then of the Xia, Shang and Zhou dynasties, to 221 B.C.—that's a span of about 2500 years. Now, if you look at the genealogical tree of Huang Di[32], (Fig.38) you will see something truly amazing: during those 2500 years every King of China was a lineal descendant of the Yellow Emperor! That means one family, broadly speaking, ruled China for 2500 years. Imagine, if you will, what the Western world would be like now if we had all been ruled by one family since well before the time of Christ. What a set-up for developing and reinforcing tradition, and thank Heaven, that the guiding concept of this civilization was virtue.

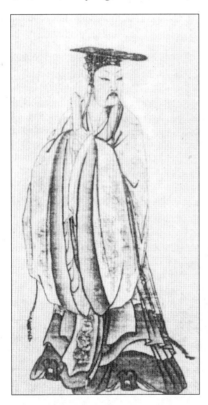

Figure 37: KING YU, THE MASTER OF THE FLOOD.

He was the last of the Sage Kings and the founder of the Xia dynasty. He was not only a consummate engineer and an exemplar of compassion, but also a shaman as indicated in footnote 48.

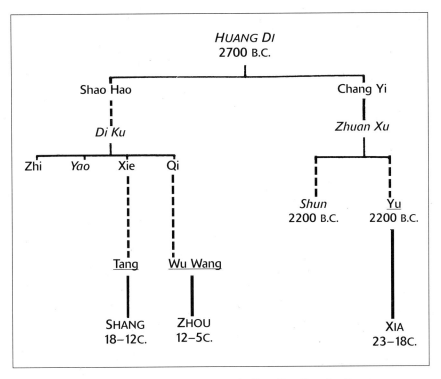

underline: Founders of Dynasties   *italics:* Five Premier Emperors

Figure 38: THE GENEALOGY OF THE YELLOW EMPEROR.
Various branches of the family tree of Huang Di were claimed as their ancestral lines by the rulers of the Xia, Shang and Zhou dynasties. Even if the claims turn out to be inaccurate, they still fostered a remarkable degree of cultural homogeneity in traditional China.

4

From Mythology to Medicine: A History of TOM

Having established the desired aura of respect for what is "traditional," I must confess that when it comes to studying the history of acupuncture, the very meaning of the word traditional itself becomes ambiguous. There are at least three different lines of tradition evolving simultaneously, and of course, continuously interacting. The most well-known is the written tradition, which consists of the relevant classics and their subsequent commentaries alongside more recently published works. A second line is the oral tradition—what is passed on from father to son, teacher to student, in a culture where this form of learning is both time-honored and the predominant mode of tuition. Finally, there is the actual historical record, unearthed by archaeologists and their ilk, which attempts to reveal the "facts" upon which the first two traditions base their teachings. As an example, both the written and the oral traditions ascribe acupuncture's *Classic of Internal Medicine* to the Yellow Emperor in the 27th century B.C., but historical studies show that this text could not have been written down until more than 2,000 years later.[33] Could it have been maintained for this long by oral transmission alone? Historical research can go only so far in documenting or rejecting parts of this, or any, oral tradition—there will always be mysteries, questions for which we have no answers, and we will see this same phenomenon happening even now in the twentieth century, in the next chapter.

Let us start with the archaeological record. The origin of acupuncture is unknown, but scholars generally agree that it was in neolithic times, at least prior to 1,000 B.C.[34] There is even some evidence to support a date as early as 3,000 B.C., the time of the Yellow Emperor himself.[35] One of the oldest Chinese books, the Classic of Mountains and Seas,[36] mentions stone needles called "bian" used to cure illness, and these same stone needles are later mentioned in the *Classic of Internal Medicine* as having originated in the East.[37] Korea is situated east of

China, and interestingly, archeological relics including stone and
bone needles putatively dated to
3000 B.C. were exavated in Korea
in 1929 and are now in their
National Museum (Fig.39). In
1963, Chinese archeologists discovered ground "bian stone" needles at a neolithic site in Inner
Mongolia (Toudaowa) which they
estimate to be between 4,000 and
10,000 years old.[38] The *Classic of
Mountains and Seas* also mentions
other needles called "zhen" in a
different context, but the ideogram
it uses for zhen is based on bamboo rather than metal, as in the
more recent ideogram for needle,
suggesting that the earliest acupuncture needles other than the bian
stones may have been of plant origin, and thus unknown to the
archaeological record.[39] Metal
acupuncture needles have been in
use at least since 800 B.C.[40], the
earliest examples being bronze needles found in 1978 in Inner
Mongolia (Dalate)[41] which are
specified only as "bronze age" and
therefore would date to the late
Xia, Shang or early Zhou dynasty
(Fig.40).

Now the archeological
record gives us some idea of the
antiquity of acupuncture, but
unfortunately it tells us little
about how acupuncture was
used or about the identity of its
practitioners. To get some
insights into these matters we
might look at the meeting of the
archaelogical and literary traditions which historically occurred

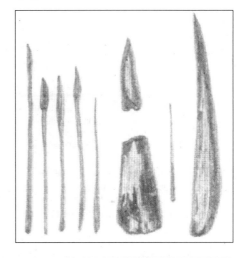

Figure 39: STONE & BONE NEEDLES.
These archeological relics from neolithic sites in Korea attest to the antiquity of
the practice of acupuncture. They were
unearthed at Songpyong-dong in 1929
and are kept in the National Museum
of Korea.

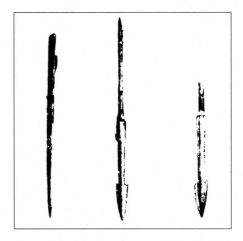

Figure 40: BRONZE NEEDLES.
These examples date from the late Zhou
dynasty, however since the "bronze age"
began as early as the Xia dynasty it is
possible that metal needles were in use
long before those in this illustration.

in two forms. The first consists of some 400 specimens of ceremonial bronze vases dating from the Xia and Shang dynasties which bear engraved inscriptions showing 1098 characers with 4200 variations.[42] This earliest strata of Chinese writing (reputed to have originated around 3,000 B.C. by Cang Xie, minister of Huang Di, The Yellow Emperor[43]) was used by the late French sinologist and acupuncturist Jacques Lavier to reconstruct the original meanings of the terms used in traditional acupuncture. His speculative interpretations have been largely ignored in scholarly circles, but are mentioned here both for

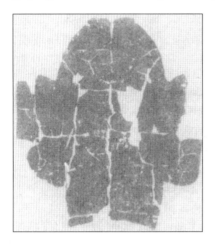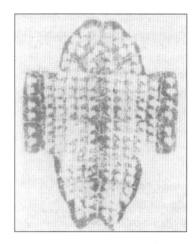

Figure 41: ORACLE BONES - A.
These Shang dynasty tortoise carapaces were used for divination, at times concerning medical issues, but mostly for affairs of state. The names of 36 diseases have so far been deciphered from them.

their intrinsic interest, and because Lavier was an important influence on J.R. Worsley as will be shown in the following chapter. The form of early Chinese writing which did seriously impact the scholarly community was that found on the so-called "oracle bones," or jiaguwen, which were only discovered in China at the beginning of the twentieth century (Fig.41). At that time farmers near Anyang in the neighborhood of the ancient capital of the Shang dynasty were selling curious pieces of inscribed bones they had dug up in their fields to drugstores as "dragon bones," a traditional component of Chinese herbal remedies. Liu Tieh-yun, a scholar who was procuring some herbal medicine to treat himself for malaria, happened to notice that the inscriptions on the dragon bones seemed to be a form of ancient writing, and after considerable research the writings were discovered to be recordings of divinations performed at the court of the kings of the Shang dynasty, whence the

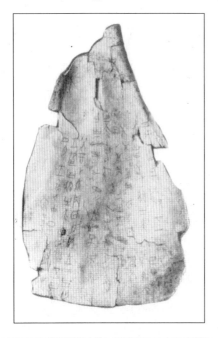

Figure 42: ORACLE BONES - B.
Carapaces and ox shoulder-blades were both used to perform and record diviniations and preserve some of the clearest examples of ancient Chinese writing. The divination itself simply involved the formation of a Y-shaped crack in response to applied heat, so large bones were often used for multiple divinations.

nickname "oracle bones."[44] The bones used were either ox shoulder blades or tortoise carapaces and plastrons which had been heated, causing cracks to appear (Fig.42). The meaning of the divination was revealed by the pattern of cracks, and both the matter to be divined and the answer given were subsequently inscribed on the cracked bone. From these records yielding about 3,000 characters[45] and from the previously mentioned bronze artifacts we have a lot of contemporary information on the nature of Shang civilization. In addition to confirming the genealogy presented in Chapter Three, the records indicate that the Shang practiced

ancestor worship in which the earliest of their line was deified as Shang Di, or "Lord on High." Illnesses in this culture were seen as punishments by angry ancestors, and the only recourse was to appease them with

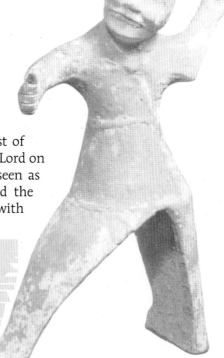

Figure 43: THE WU OR SHAMAN.
This dancing ceramic figure is from approximately the third century A.D., probably from the Luoyang district. Shamanism had a strong influence on Daoism, and through it on TOM.

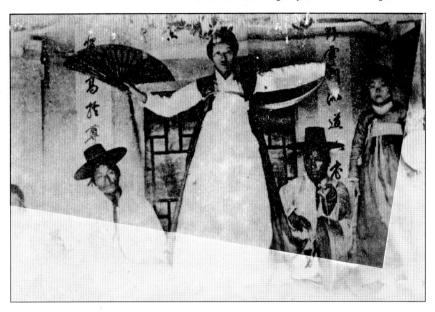

Figure 44: A KOREAN MANSHIN.
This female shaman was photographed during her ritual "dance" near the turn of the century. Essentially identical ceremonies can still be observed in present day Korea.

the proper rituals and sacrificial offerings. For this, a specialist was needed, the shaman, or as he was called in Chinese, the wu (Fig.43). Thus the earliest type of medical practice in China of which we have knowledge is a form of shamanism in which the wu divined the will of the deceased Spirits and then carried out a ritual to appease them. This type of shamanism is indeed native to an extensive northern hemispheric zone centered in the Altai—Ural mountains including Manchuria and Mongolia in China, and also Siberia, and its practice has amazingly continued to this day with only relatively minor alterations in Korea, where the shaman is called mu or mudang or manshin instead of wu (Fig.44). Archeological digs in Shensi Province, the cradle of Chinese civilization, have yielded artifacts dating to the Xia dynasty side by side with Siberian pottery, indicating the antiquity of shamanistic cultural influence on China.[46] Also, the similarity of the Chinese and Native American shamanistic healers, or medicine men[47], begins to make my facetious remarks in Chapter Three on the origins of acupuncture approach the domain of credible hypothesis, for as we shall see, the earliest acupuncturists may very well have been the shamen.

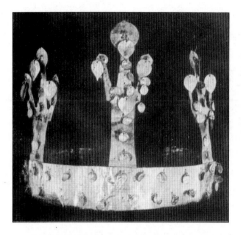

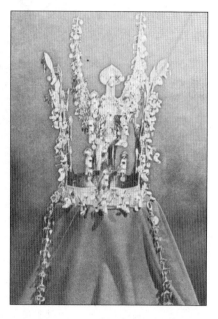

Figure 45: THE COSMIC TREE.
Shamanistic crowns discovered in Korea invariably contain tree-shaped ornaments alluding to the central axis of the cosmos, along which the shaman could fly in ecstatic trance.

Many of the cardinal ideas of TOM can be found in shamanism, starting with the doctrine of the trinity of Heaven, Earth and Man. In its earliest form, the three realms were Heaven, Earth and the Underworld represented by a cosmic tree with its roots in the Underworld, its trunk on Earth and its branches in Heaven (Fig. 45). The shaman was the one individual who could, in ecstatic trance, fly up to Heaven or down to the Underworld to commune with the Spirits and intercede for his community so as to restore harmony. Thus, it is not strange to find that in the earliest traditions, the shaman was the king, who as the "Son of Heaven" was the only individual allowed to perform the rites to Heaven and Earth, and was described as the "one man."[48] Eventually the

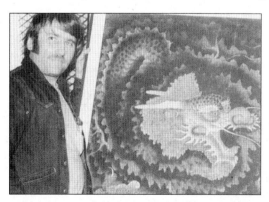

Figure 46: THE RAIN-BRINGING DRAGON.
This painting is the largest surviving depiction of its kind in Korea, and since its successful use in the Los Angeles drought in 1977 it has resided in the Emileh Museum of Folk Art in Korea. Noted author Alan Covell is seen unpacking the painting at the museum's inauguration in Songni-san.

roles of king and shaman became separated in China and over many hundreds of years the shaman was reduced to a much lower social status, but not before leaving his mark on the concept of illness and recovery. I've used the masculine gender in referring to the shaman because apparently the early shaman-kings were male, but as the two roles became distinct sometime before 1,000 B.C., the wu became predominantly female as are the mudang still active in Korea today. The Chinese character for wu, 巫 , depicts two shamen dancing to obtain rain, and forms part of the more complex characters for both divination (shi 筮, where the Yarrow-Achillea stalks used in *Yi Jing* consultation are included) and spiritual power (ling 靈 depicting the dancers calling out for rain). As recently as 1977 a Korean shamanist ritual was employed to deal with the drought in Los Angeles which had lasted one hundred days at that point. Following the ceremony which involved the ritual use of the rain-bearing dragon painting in Figure 46 a cloud burst occurred within hours![49]

I've gotten a little side-tracked in terms of the history of acupuncture, but it turns out that as I've just said, the wu were probably very important in this regard, possibly even being the first acupuncturists. The *Shuo Wen Jie Zi*, an early Chinese dictionary, identified the first doctor as a sorcerer or wu, named Pan.[50] Paul Unschuld has pointed out that the development of medical thought in China went through several stages, and that ancestor worship was succeeded by demonology in which frankly evil spirits (xie guei) were now identified as the cause of illnesses, and the shaman's job expanded to include exorcism. For this role the wu employed spears and other sharp weapons to drive out the demons. Of course we do not know that those pointed objects were ever applied to or inserted into the patient's body, but it is curious that the oldest Chinese character for medicine or physician, yi, depicted the wu over which are drawn a quiver of arrows on the left and a spear on the right, (毉) possibly alluding to a primitive form of

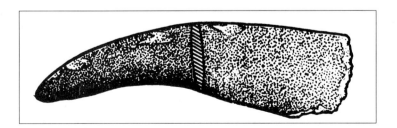

Figure 47: A CHINESE BIAN STONE NEEDLE.
This "bian" from a Shang dynasty site at Taixi is called a "stone hook."
Compare its shape to that of the appendages in Figures 48 and 49.

acupuncture.[51] It has even been asserted that fragments of the divinatory carapaces excavated along with the oracle bones were sometimes formed in the shape of needles, and were used to perform acupuncture as early as three thousand years ago.[52] Another suggestive connection is that the earliest artifacts claimed as acupuncture needles, made of stone and fishbone, were excavated in Korea where the shamanistic tradition has been most clearly documented. A final piece of evidence possibly supporting the wu as the first acupuncturists is the claim that the first acupuncture points used were the "thirteen ghost points" which are classically recommended for demonic possession, or what would now be described as mental illness of one sort or another. Although the specification of which points were to be used seems to date to the Tang dynasty, it is traditionally claimed that they were discovered or at least used by Bian Que, one of the first acupuncturists whose name we know.[53] Figure 47 shows a "hook-shaped" stone artifact excavated from a Shang dynasty tomb at Taixi (Hubei Province) in 1973. It was contained in a protective leather casket and is identified by Chinese archaeologists as a "bian" stone needle. Figure 48 shows a crown from one of the ancient shaman-kings of Silla (Korea) which interestingly also has "hook-shaped" stone (jade) attachments (kokok) (Fig.49).

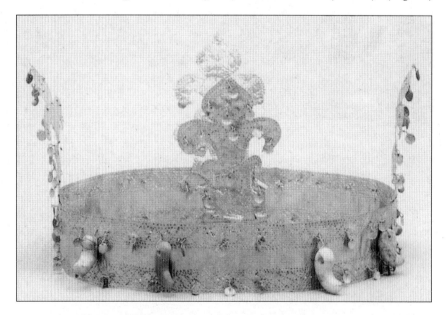

Figure 48: KAYA GOLD CROWN.
This Korean shaman's crown from around the fifth century A.D. contains numerous jade stone hook-shaped ornaments, called "kokok," similar in form to the "bian" in Figure 47.

These are said to be representative of tiger claws and thus symbolically would impart their power as weapons[54], but noting the similarity in appearance of the "bian" stones and the "kokok" stones, I would like to suggest as a further hypothesis that these "tiger claws" might have originally been used as "bian" needles by the early shamen.

It was only in the later Zhou dynasty that the character "yi" for physician was changed, with an alcoholic extract (yu) being substituted for the dancing shamen (wu) who were slipping in social status.[55] Interestingly, in English the alcoholic beverages which replaced the shaman in the character for physician are colloquially referred to as "spirits." The wu have left a considerable legacy in traditional acupuncture. Their spiritual power (ling) became the axis of *The Canon of Acupuncture*, the original title of the second half of the *Nei Jing* now known as the *Ling Shu* (*Spiritual Pivot*). I should also point out that there is only a hazy distinction between much of Shamanism and Daoism, especially religious Daoism, which superceeded it in China, whereas its direct offshoot in Japan, Shintoism, has maintained a strong shamanistic character[56], but I'm getting ahead of myself in this historical narrative. The main idea which I'd like to emphasize as being carried over from shamanism to

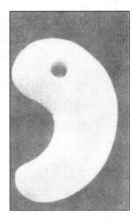

Figure 49: KOKOK.
These shamanistic symbols, used by the royalty in Korea have also been found on royal jewelry in Japan where they are called magatama. Scholars have so far been unable to agree upon the meaning of these decorations, and the author offers the hypothesis that they might be symbolic of the bian stone needles used by the shamen in their role as the originators of acupuncture.

traditional acupuncture is the central importance of the Spirit in all matters of health and illness. Along with it go the twin themes of purification and exorcism which, although later given less attention, were never absent from the practice of acupuncture until developments in the twentieth century. It should come as no surprise therefore, that coincident with the despiritualization of acupuncture in Communist China, was the outlawing of shamanism in North Korea in 1950.[57]

Let us return, then, to an examination of the literary tradition in which acupuncture is first mentioned very briefly in several anecdotes about the doctors Yi Yuan and Bian Que in works compiled only towards the end of the Zhou and the beginning of the Han dynasties. Clearly these stories, which I will recount in discussing the careers of these two famous acupuncturists are not very helpful in understanding the origins of acupuncture. Therefore, I shall start by discussing the classical medical texts, beginning with the *Yellow Emperor's Classic of Internal Medicine*, or *Nei Jing*, as I will now refer to it, for convenience. Written sometime prior to 100 B.C., it is the earliest book that is overtly about acupuncture, but to truly understand its philosophical concepts, which underlie traditional acupuncture, we must look further back, to the *Classic of Changes*, or *Yi Jing*, whose date is likewise controversial, but probably as early as 1100 B.C.[58]

The *Yi Jing* is most commonly known as a book for divination, and indeed it had that ancient usage. The diagrams it contains were supposedly discovered by Emperor Fu Xi, one of China's legendary Culture Heroes, who was said to have lived sometime prior to 3,000 B.C., and who is also said to have discovered the use of nets for hunting and fishing[59] (Fig.50). The diagrams in the *Yi Jing* consist of the eight trigrams and 64 hexagrams whose permutations represent the continuous process of change which we experience in every aspect of nature (Fig.51). Fu Xi was reputedly inspired to think of the original eight trigrams following a vision he had of a "dragon-horse" emerging from the Yellow River with a design on its back, called the He Tu or River Diagram (Fig.52). This diagram, and the eight trigrams it inspired, contain the essence upon which all later traditional Chinese medical thought is based. Starting from a reverence for the transcendent power of numbers themselves, these diagrams are the foundation of the two organizing principles of traditional acupuncture—the theories of Yin-Yang and the Five Elements.[60] The trigrams are made up of broken and solid lines, symbolizing Yin and Yang respectively, and like the binary code used in computer language to which they are equivalent, they can be

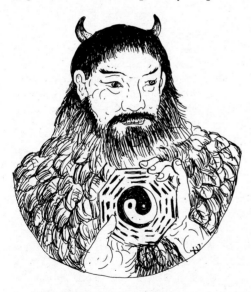

Figure 50: Fu Xi.
This legendary emperor (note the horns) was reputed to have lived prior to 3,000 B.C. He was the first of the Culture Heroes, and is shown holding the symbol of the eight trigrams, although the sequence depicted is a garbled version of the one with which he is usually associated.

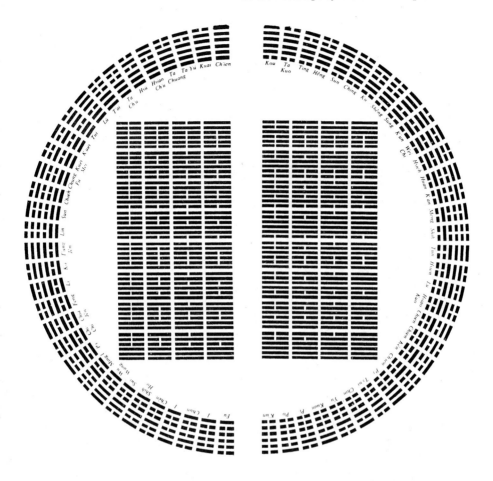

Figure 51: THE 64 HEXAGRAMS.
These figures, which make up the *Yi Jing* or Classic of Changes, are arranged in a circular and a square formation inspired by Fu Xi and articulated by Shao Yung in the eleventh century A.D.

used to represent an infinite variety of information. The Five Element theory is implicit in both the River diagram and in certain arrangements of the trigrams, and it is also applicable to all the manifestations of variety in the universe, but has no obvious analogy in modern Western thought. What is common to both Yin-Yang and Five Element theories is the assumption that reality is nothing more nor less than "matter-energy" in a continuous process of motion and change. As I have already indicated, the Chinese word for this matter-energy is Qi, which is often simply translated as energy, but strictly speaking, denotes a very subtle substance making up the human organism, Man, and also all the

10,000 things in creation. It is by influencing the Qi with needles inserted into the body, that the traditional acupuncturist attempts to restore a normal harmonious state of functioning, using either or both Yin-Yang and Five Element theories of energetics, as a guide.

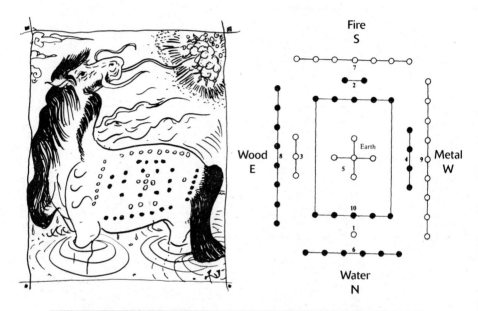

Figure 52: THE HE TU OR RIVER DIAGRAM.
Although no ancient records exist depicting the He Tu, its form and numerical relationships have been described as pictured above at least since the Song dynasty.

Following Fu Xi was another legendary emperor, Shen Nong, who is credited with being the father of herbal medicine and agriculture, and also with the invention of the plow (Fig.53). He is reputed to have gained his knowledge by self-experimentation, in which he poisoned himself up to eighty times a day, but was able to recover by relying on his previously acquired herbal knowledge.[61] His ability to survive these experiments was also legendarily attributed to two "magical powers." The first was the possession of a magical whisk which revealed if plants were poisonous or not, and also disclosed their nature. The second was the possession of a transparent body that allowed him to see how each herb affected the different parts inside his body. If an organ became poisoned, he could see it, and neutralize the poison merely by rubbing the affected part with the appropriate antidote.[62] Herbal medicine is considered by some to be an older component of traditional Oriental medicine than is acupuncture, though it was first mentioned on bamboo slips dating to the late Zhou dynasty. While it is based on both the Yin-Yang and Five Element theories inherent in the *Yi Jing*, it has had its own line of development that at times has paralleled that of acupuncture, and at other times has been quite divergent. This situation has created a good deal of controversy and confusion that has continued into modern times, and will be mentioned again and again as this story unfolds. Shen Nong is honorarily credited with writing the first book about herbs, *Shen Nong's Pharmacopeia*, however, this is an obvious anachronism, as is the attribution of the *Yi Jing* to Fu Xi.[63] In the same manner, the Yellow Emperor, who followed Shen Nong, did not actually write the *Nei Jing* (Fig.54).

Fu Xi, Shen Nong and Huang Di are referred to as the Three Culture Heroes. We can see the rubric of the Three Powers operating through them in the Chinese conception of their own historical development. Fu Xi exemplifies the virtue of Heaven, being the source of norms or guidelines as seen abstractly in the formative trigrams or more concretely in the nets whose lines catch things instead of concepts. Shen Nong exemplifies the virtue of Earth by his observations on the different types of soil and how to cultivate the five types of cereal grains using the plow and other agricultural implements and by the use of plants for healing. With Huang Di, the Yellow Emperor, the virtue of Man becomes manifest, and history proper begins. He is credited with introducing writing, acupuncture and the systematic use of family names. Prior to the Yellow Emperor, what family names there were contained the radical[64] for woman, suggesting a matriarchal society, but the Yellow Emperor was himself an exception to this rule, his surname being Gongsun, or Duke's Grandson[65], suggesting a transition to the subsequently dominant patriarchal society. The time of the Yellow Emperor's reign historically corresponds to the transition in neolithic cultures from the earlier

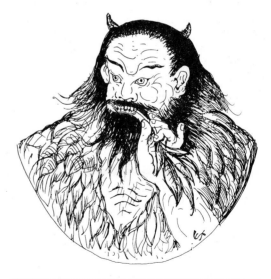

Figure 53: SHEN NONG.
Another legendary (horned) emperor who came after Fu Xi and before Huang Di, Shen Nong is considered the father of herbal medicine. He is depicted tasting an herb to determine its properties.

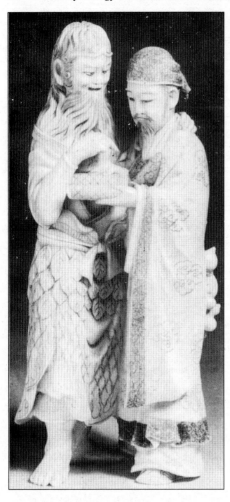

Figure 54: HUANG DI AND SHEN NONG.
This ivory carving shows the founders of the two main branches of TOM, acupuncture and herbalism, discussing medical scripture. Once again, Shen Nong on the left (note the leaves on his clothing) has an other-wordly appearance, while Huang Di on the right has a perfectly normal human form.

Yang Shao, based on matriarchal fertility rites which peaked around 3,000 B.C., to the later Lung Shan, who introduced patriarchal ancestor worship as recorded on their oracle bones and whose culture peaked around 2,000 B.C.[66] Living in an age which straddled both cultures, the Yellow Emperor was the natural choice of patron for a system of medicine which sought to keep a balance between the masculine and feminine principles (i.e.: Yang and Yin). It is also fitting that the emperors signifying the virtues of Heaven and Earth should remain legendary, while the Yellow Emperor, signifying the virtue of Man, is the proper starting point for His story (history).

As related in Chapter Three, after the epoch of the Five Premier Emperors[67] ushered in by Huang Di, came that of the Sage Kings, Yao, Shun and Yu, and their struggles with the great flood. Like Fu Xi before him, Yu was also aided by a vision of a miraculous animal. In his case, it was a "divine" tortoise, who emerged from the Luo River with a numerical design on its back which came to be known as the Luo Shu or Luo scroll (Fig.55). This design is a pictorial model of the numerological curiosity called the magic square, which adds up to 15 in all directions. It is considered to be the graphic form of the "Great Plan" described in the *Classic of History* which includes perhaps the earliest reference in Chinese literature to the Five Elements and their associated numbers. The tortoise itself is a highly

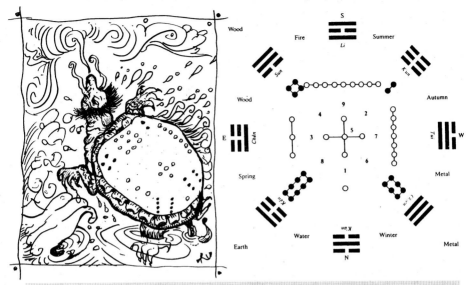

Figure 55: THE LUO SHU OR LUO SCROLL.
Like the He Tu, the form of the Luo Shu was apparently specified only in the Song dynasty, as no ancient depictions exist. It is often shown simply as a "magic square" adding up to 15 in all directions.

symbolic animal, whose back is round like Heaven and whose bottom is square and flat like Earth—it's a representation of the microcosm. Thus it is not surprising that its shell was used for divination, producing some of the "oracle bones" mentioned previously.

Following the Sage Kings were the Three Dynasties: Xia, Shang and Zhou. I've presented the more that 2500 year time-span up to this point with an emphasis on its homogeneity as a way of highlighting the context within which traditional Oriental medical thought arose, but actually, the birth of the classical texts on acupuncture and herbal medicine came towards the end of, or shortly after, the most contentious phase of Chinese history, in the latter days of the Zhou dynasty, known as both the Warring States period (403-221 B.C.) and as that of the "Hundred Schools of Thought" (551-233 B.C.). These schools all influenced to one degree or another, the development of the framework for traditional acupuncture, and are thus important to mention.

Foremost, of course, is Daoism, which like its offshoot Oriental medicine proper, took the Yellow Emperor for its patron, while its canon was the *Way and Its Virtue* by Lao Zi, whose ideas were further developed by Zhuang Zi and others[68] (Figs.56, 57). The Dao or Way, its central concept, can be thought of as the ineffable unity of nature that we can experience, but can never adequately describe. Daoists are of two sorts, the philosophical school, or Dao Jia[69], whose members,

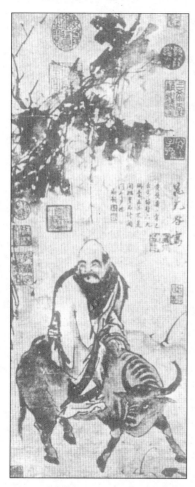

Figure 56: LAO ZI.
The founder of Daoism and author of *The Way and its Virtue (Dao De Jing)*, Lao Zi is often depicted riding a water buffalo on his departure from China towards an unknown destination in the West.

starting with Lao Zi, contributed to the fundamental assumptions underlying traditional acupuncture, and the religious group, or Dao Jiao,[70] which emerged later and had a stronger influence on the development of herbal medicine, based on their experiences in searching for elixirs of longevity and immortality. Daoist temples are called "guan," whose original meaning was "to look, especially to observe natural phenomena in order to divine the future"[71]. It seems to me that the Daoists of both groups were unique in their ability to harmoniously combine the roles of scientist and mystic, a combination at once powerful and yet charming. They were equally at home with philosophical conceptualizations such as Yin-Yang and the Five Elements as with physiological conceptualizations such as essence (Jing), vital energy (Qi) and spirit (Shen), the Three Treasures that form the basis for the sexual, gymnastic and respiratory yogas that they devised for the return to the oneness of the Dao. They stressed non-interference with nature (wu wei) and the principle of learning by experience, not by authority[72]—both important teachings in traditional acupuncture.

While the Daoists were noted for their avoidance of court-life, the Naturalists, who in many other ways resembled them, were anxious to serve as court advisors. They were, in large part, responsible for the development of the major theoretical concepts of Oriental medicine, the Yin-Yang and Five Element theories, which they originally used in a political context. Yin-Yang theory provided a basis for the court diviners to interpret the oracles of the *Yi Jing* while Zou Yen[73] (c. 350–270 B.C.) used the theory of the Five Elements to interpret the pattern of succession of ruling dynasties, a subject of great interest to those in positions of power. Zou Yen's followers, the

Naturalists, called themselves the Yin-Yang Jia, or School of Yin-Yang, reflecting the close connection between Yin-Yang and Five Element theories in the formative period of traditional acupuncture, a lesson to be kept in mind when contemplating the rift between partisans of these two paradigms which emerged in the twentieth century. Both Yin-Yang and Five Element theories are expressions of correlative thinking, a way of looking at the universe in which "conceptions are not subsumed under one another, but placed side by side in a pattern and in which things influence one another not by acts of mechanical causation but by a kind of inductance."[74] Learning to think inductively, to look for patterns rather than causal agents, is one of the major tasks in mastering traditional acupuncture, and involves a kind of cognitive shift that can be difficult for those growing up in the Western scientific culture. This inductive mode of thought is no less scientific than the deductive mode we are used to, and as Joseph Needham observed, "Chinese coordinative thinking was not primitive thinking in the sense that it was an alogical or pre-logical chaos in which anything could be the cause of anything else . . . It was a picture of an extremely and precisely ordered universe in which things "fitted" so exactly that you could not insert a hair between them."[75]

The naturalist philosophers were not alone in their desire for positions of influence as state advisors. The most famous Chinese philosopher of all time, Confucius, who was born in 552 B.C., spent his whole life looking for a feudal prince who would put into practice his teachings, which were based on a return to the ways of the ancient kings (Fig.58). Thus, the hallmark of Confucianism was its emphasis on tradition, and in this we can appreciate its potential importance in the development of "traditional" acupuncture. The Confucian school was known as the Ju Jia or school of Scholars, and Confucius himself is associated with the Five Classics, though whether he edited them or simply used them in his teaching is open to dispute. His focus was on human behavior, his stance was a moral one, and his ideal was the "jun zi" or superior man, one who embodied the moral

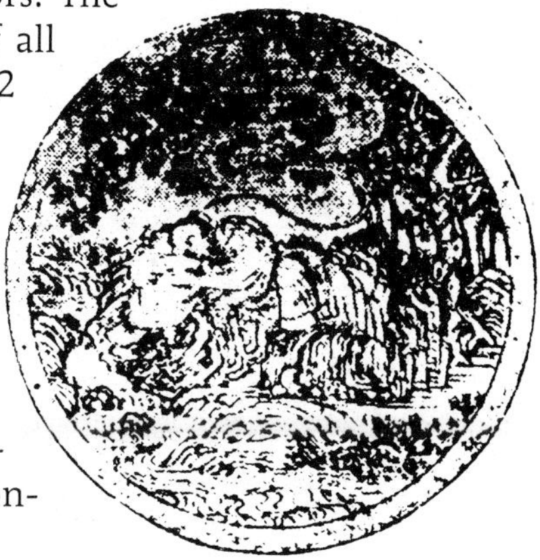

Figure 57: ZHUANG ZI.
Second only to Lao Zi in his fame as a proponent of philosophical Daoism, Zhuang Zi is best known for his thought-provoking tales. His image fades into ambiguity in this wood carving, reminiscent of the Yin/Yang symbol itself, shown in Figure 80.

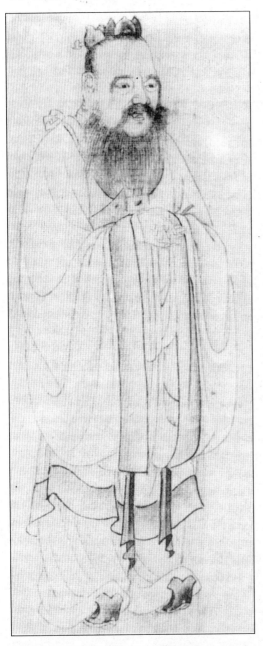

Figure 58: CONFUCIUS.
The most well-known of all Chinese philosophers, Confucius claimed he was only a transmitter of tradition, ways handed down from the ancient kings.

virtues including li (ritual or decorum), ren (humanity), yi (righteousness or propriety), zhi (wisdom), xin (trustworthiness), cheng (loyalty), xiao (filial piety) and cheng (sincerity).[76]

In summarizing the teachings of these three philosophical schools of the Warring States period, whose teachings were the principal ones to survive in traditional Chinese culture, we once again encounter the imagery of the Three Powers. The Daoists were concerned with the intangible Dao, a Heavenly concept of the ultimate guiding reality, while the Naturalists focused on its Earthly projection in the form of the concrete laws of Yin/Yang and the Five Elements. The Confucians, representative of the "middle way," focused on the level of Man, and these three together evolved a complete and harmonious description of the universe which provided the intellectual basis for the development of traditional Oriental medicine and acupuncture. There were other philosophies that developed into schools of thought during the Warring States period, including the Legalists (Fa Jia), Logicians (Ming Jia), and Utilitarians (Mo Jia), but as these had much less of an impact on the development of medical thought, we will skip over them.

Returning to the Warring States period, it was during this time that the first book about acupuncture, the *Nei Jing*, was written. From this point on, the oral and written traditions of acupuncture became distinct entities. The doctors of higher status were referred to as Ju Yi[77] or scholar physicians, who gained their knowledge mostly from books, while the less prestigious doctors were called Shi Yi[78], or genealogical physicians, whose skills were transmitted from father to son, and who frequently practiced as itinerants, whence their nickname, Ling Yi or bell ringers.[79] This difference in status interestingly had no reliable correlation with the practitioner's level of skill, as there were famous physicians from both traditions throughout history.[80] All traditional acupuncturists, however, accept the *Nei Jing* as the canon on which their practice is based, although there is still some dispute as to whether it was a product of the late Warring States period or the early Han dynasty. It is written in the form of a series of dialogs between the Yellow Emperor and his medical advisors, one of whom (Qi Bo) gives the following account of the origin of the traditional Oriental diagnostic principles (Fig.59):

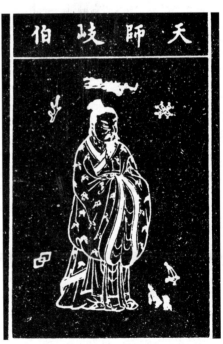

"Color and pulse are valued by Shang Di, and they were taught by the teachers of former times. In ancient times, a teacher by the name of Jiudai Ji was entrusted with the task of systematizing colors and pulses and researching into the secrets of the manifestations of Spirit; he then discovered the Five Elements . . . the four seasons, the eight winds and the six directions which follow a regular pattern to which colors and pulses correspond . . . To know the essential aspects of diagnosis, one should start with colors and pulses."[81]

Figure 59: QI BO.
The most prominent advisor of the Yellow Emperor in the *Nei Jing*, Qi Bo is referred to as a Heavenly Master, having studied the medical treatment of patients from two generations prior to his own.

Now Shang Di or Lord on High, was the ancestral deity worshipped as I have indicated by the shaman-kings of the Shang dynasty—thus the principles of acupuncture and Oriental medical theory can be seen as having evolved from early shamanistic practices, as had the very character for physician, yi. When the Yellow Emperor stated that, "in ancient times diseases were cured by prayers alone . . . but nowadays physicians treat disease with herbs internally and with acupuncture externally"[82] he was most likely recounting the specific evolution of shamanistic practices over time.

Considering therapeutics, the *Nei Jing* already emphasizes the medical skills including acupuncture and herbal prescription, which I am hypothesizing as having developed from the earlier shamanistic spiritual practices.[83] The *Nei Jing* does not, however, give equal attention to acupuncture and herbal medicine, but predominantly deals with the former. References to physicians in the Chinese literature prior to the *Nei Jing* (with the exception of Yu Fu) tended to mention acupuncture and herbal medicine together, as in the stories of Yi Yuan and Bian Que which follow, so the divergence of acupuncture and herbal medicine seems to be an accompaniment of the formation of a separate literary tradition which then followed its own line of development. Yu Fu, considered to be a contemporary of Qi Bo, is an interesting exception to the above rule, in that he is specifically mentioned as having used acupuncture and moxibustion but not herbal medicine. Some have concluded from this that he was the first true acupuncture specialist (Fig.60).

Yi Yuan is related to have gone to treat the Prince of Chin in 580 B.C., but found his disease to be incurable and said, "no needle can penetrate it, no drug can reach it."[84] The Prince of Guo, sometime between the fourth and sixth century B.C., although lying deathlike in a coma, was more fortunate. His doctor, Bian Que, revived him with acupuncture, and then completed his cure with moxibustion and herb tea[85] (Fig.61). Bian Que figures in several other legendary tales related variously by Si Ma Qian, Han Feizi and Liezi. In the most astonishing one he is reported to have performed the first, and probably only, exchange transplant of the human heart between two patients who were each anesthetized for three days with a magical liquor.[86] Another tale relates how he prognosticated the development of a mortal illness in King Yuan of Cai while the latter was still totally asymptomatic, and how despite Bian Que's warnings, the King refused to admit he was sick until it was too late for treatment, and he died as predicted. It is often said that Bian Que was the first to systematize the four methods of examination and he is also legendarily credited with authorship of the *Nan Jing* (*Classic of Difficulties*) but this assertion at least can be rejected because the *Nan Jing* is a much later work. Bian Que was unfortunately assassinated on orders from the medical bureaucracy,[87] the sad fate of many a visionary, but because of his unsurpassed technical skills

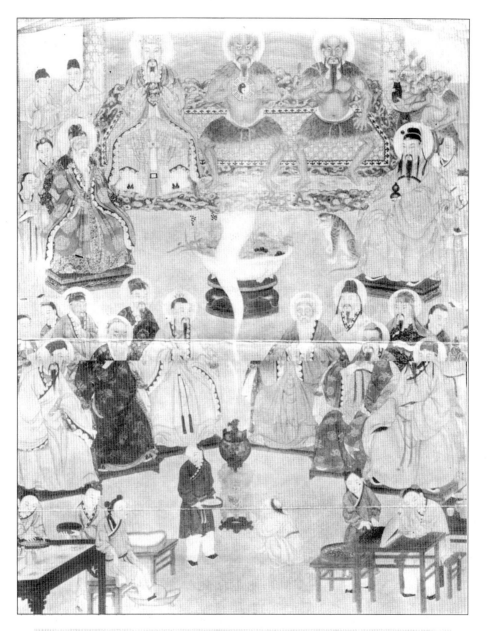

Figure 60: A Galaxy of Notables in Chinese Medicine.

This painting, reproduced in Hume, is said to contain the following individuals, although their identities are not clearly indicated in several cases: Huang Di, Fu Xi, Shen Nong, Qi Bo, Yu Fu, Sun Si-miao, Bian Que, Ma Shi-huang, Zhang Zhong-jing, Hua Tuo, Zhang Dao-ling, Chunyu Yi, Ge Hong and Huang-fu Mi. Generally they are the major figures sequentially from left to right and from top to bottom although the individual to the right of Sun Si-miao is skipped. The only individual in this list not described elsewhere in this book is Ma Shi-huang who was a legendary veterinarian during the reign of Huang Di, famous for treating horses, and who once cured a sick dragon with acupuncture!

combined with a whole-hearted dedication to the care of his patients, Bian Que has been revered by the Chinese as the "Father of Medicine" and his birthday, the 28th day of the fourth lunar month is celebrated as a national holiday.

Moxibustion, the therapeutic technique of burning Artemisia tinder (moxa or ai) on or above the skin is also less intensively discussed than is acupuncture in the *Nei Jing*, but because the systematics of its use are so similar to those of acupuncture, this has caused much less in the way of doctrinal splits than has the parallel development of herbal medicine and acupuncture. Moxibustion is probably as ancient a practice as is acupuncture, and was mentioned by both Zhuang Zi[88] and Mencius[89] (Fig.62). Naturally, the archaeological record is less helpful here than in the case of acupuncture, but the discovery in 1973 of silk books from prior to the third century B.C. in the tombs near Ma wang dui village in Hunan Province included two treatises concerning moxibustion along Meridian pathways that are of a much more primitive stage of systematization than is found in the *Nei Jing*.

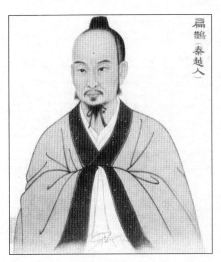

Figure 61: BIAN QUE (407-310 B.C.)
Revered by the Chinese as the "Father of Medicine," he was proficient in the use of acupuncture, moxibustion and herbs.

This has led some scholars to suggest that moxibustion was developed prior to acupuncture, but I would like to propose a variation on this hypothesis: from what I have described so far, it is likely that acupuncture originated from the shamanistic tradition still extant to the east of China in present-day Korea. Moxibustion on the other hand, might have developed separately in China as part of the doctrine of systematic as opposed to magical correspondence, and these two traditions later met and were integrated into a coherent approach. Such an interpretation is supported by Lavier's reconstruction of the origin of traditional Chinese medical thought mentioned earlier, which is based on the idea that the original conceptualizations of systematic correspondence, typified by the doctrine of the Five Elements were developed by a Protochinese agrarian civilization, and that the mysterious forces which more closely fit a paradigm of magical correspondence, were actually a later addition, introduced into Chinese

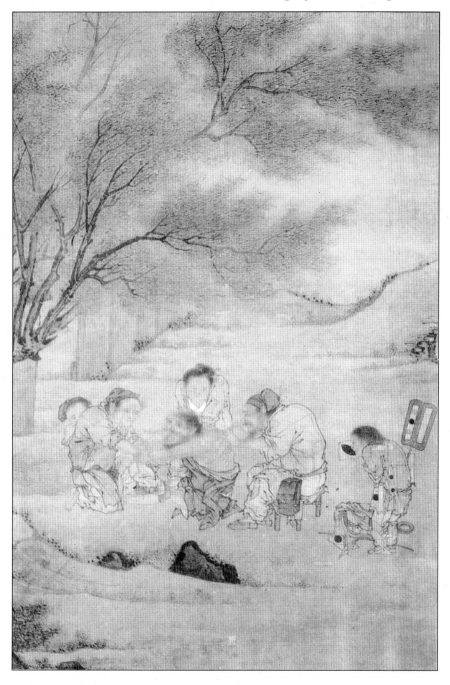

Figure 62: MOXIBUSTION.
This painting by Li Tang of the Song dynasty depicts a village doctor applying moxa. The painful technique of direct scarring moxibustion is now generally replaced by gentler non-scarring techniques.

medical thought by the waves of nomadic invaders from the shamanistic cultures around these Protochinese farmers. This hypothesis is also consistent with the traditional origin of the different therapeutic techniques of Oriental medicine which was given in the *Nei Jing* according to the following five part correlative scheme: stone needle acupuncture in the East to treat ulcers and abscesses, herbal medicine in the West to treat internal diseases, moxibustion in the North to treat diseases due to cold, fine needle acupuncture in the south to treat rheumatic diseases and massage, breathing and physical exercises in the Center to treat paralytic diseases.[90]

In addition to presenting historical material on diagnostics and therapeutics, the *Nei Jing* contains voluminous theoretical and practical information on all the different aspects of traditional Oriental medicine, tying them together into a seamless whole in such a thorough and elevated manner that it is still treated as the "Bible." We don't know who actually compiled the *Nei Jing*, but undoubtedly, it was a group effort with numerous revisions. It consists of two parts, *Su Wen* (*Simple Questions*) and *Ling Shu* (*Spiritual Pivot*) of 81 chapters each. *Su Wen* is primarily about fundamental theory, while *Ling Shu* is primarily about the practice of acupuncture and was originally called *Zhen Jing* (*Acupuncture Classic*) prior to the seventh century A.D. The standard edition in use today dates to 762 A.D., when it was compiled by Wang Bing-ci, who is believed to have added at least seven chapters of his own to replace those already lost by his time.[91]

Closely connected to the *Nei Jing* in both time and spirit is the *Nan Jing*[92] or *Classic of Difficulties*, probably written in the first century A.D.[93] and again of unknown authorship, although as mentioned, it has spuriously been attributed to Bian Que. It derives its name from the fact that it is composed of a series of 81 (!) questions and answers about unresolved issues in the *Nei Jing*. One of the cardinal issues that it tackles is that of the proper assignment of positions on the radial artery for the pulses of the twelve main Organs and Meridians, which assignment is used in performing "pulse diagnosis," the most important diagnostic method in traditional acupuncture. From the pulse, the acupuncturist gleans information about the functioning of all the components of the human organism, and from sequential readings, can tell if the patient's health is improving or not in response to treatment. The version of the pulse positions given in the *Nan Jing* is not the only one considered to be correct by traditional acupuncturists, but it was the one which spread to other countries early on, and thus forms the basis for the styles of acupuncture taught and practiced most widely in Japan, Korea and the West.[94] The major alternative set of assignments which were proposed over one thousand years later, in the Ming dynasty (1368–1644) are by contrast the ones which became the predominant traditional teaching in China and this divergence of traditions has been a source of confusion that has continued into the present[95] (Fig.63).

In discussing these early Classics, we've crossed from the Warring states Period (480–220 B.C.) of the Zhou dynasty to the Han dynasty (202 B.C.–220 A.D.) without mentioning the intervening, though brief Qin dynasty (221 B.C.–207 B.C.) which was a time of massive change in China. It was the only time the proponents of the Legalist school (Fa Jia), the least humane of the different philosophies, had the dominant voice in government. In their struggle to overturn the traditional beliefs of their adversaries, they ordered the burning of all books except those having to do with divination, agriculture and

	Left wrist		A	Right wrist	
Distal:	Small Intestine	Heart		Lung	Large Intestine
Middle:	Gall Bladder	Liver		Spleen	Stomach
Proximal:	Bladder	Kidneys		Life Gate	Three Heater

	Superficial	Deep	B	Deep	Superficial
Distal:	Pericardium	Heart		Lungs	Sternum
Middle:	Gall Bladder	Liver		Spleen	Stomach
Proximal:	Large Intestine Bladder	Kidney		Kidney	Three Heater Life Gate Small Intestine

Figure 63: PULSE POSITIONS

(A) shows the Han dynasty assignments common to the *Nan Jing* (c. 100-200) and *Mai Jing* (280). The pulse in the deep position at the proximal location on the right wrist was redesignated as the Pericardium at least as early as the Yuan dynasty, and is taught as such by the inheritors of this tradition (i.e. the Five Element schools including LA) today. This distinction is of minor practical consequence since the meridian pathway for both Life Gate and Pericardium has been identical, the Hand Jue Yin Meridian, since the *Nan Jing*. (B) shows the Ming dynasty assignments from *Zhang Jie-bing's Complete Book* (1624) which are the basis for the teachings about the pulse incorporated in TCM at present. It is based on morphologic considerations (material) rather than the Five Element (energetic) considerations found in A. This figure is based on material in Kaptchuk-1 (p. 300), Mann-1 (p. 133) and Birch (p. 4).

medicine. Thus, the development of acupuncture was fortunately less affected than most other aspects of Chinese life by the "fires of Qin." The other event for which the Qin dynasty is both famous and infamous was the building of the Great Wall, an undertaking completed at enormous human expense. The Chinese themselves have always viewed the Qin dynasty with extreme distaste,[96] so without further ado let us return to the ensuing Han dynasty.

Aside from the bronze needles recently discovered in Inner Mongolia, the earliest metal acupuncture needles excavated by archeologists of which I am aware were found in the tomb of Liu Sheng who was the elder brother of Han dynasty Emperor Wu dating to 113 B.C. Four gold and five silver needles were recovered from the tomb in Hebei province in 1968, and the better preserved gold ones are shown in Figure 64.

There were several famous doctors in the Han dynasty who left their stamp on traditional acupuncture. Chunyu Yi[97] (born in 216 B.C.) had his biography included in the *Historical Records* primarily because of his meticulous defense in 154 B.C. against an accusation of malpractice, which defense was preserved in court records and then relayed to us by Si Ma Qian (Fig.65). In it, Chunyu Yi related 25 clinical case histories from his practice, based on detailed records that he kept of each of the patients he treated. These records enabled him to estimate his percentage of successes and failures, and thus find a guide

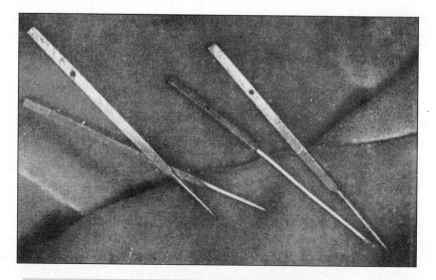

Figure 64: GOLD NEEDLES.
These needles from the Han dynasty show vastly improved workmanship compared to the Zhou dynasty bronze needles pictured in Figure 40.

to more accurate treatment. For this he became known as the "father of case histories."[98] However, it was his description of the advice he received from his teacher, Yang Qing, to throw away his "recipe books" (fang shu) and follow instead the *Pulse Treatise of Huang Di and Bian Que* that makes his story most relevant for present day practitioners who are still divided over the issue of "formula" versus "energetic" treatment. Yang Qing had tutored Chunyu Yi for three years in the techniques of pulse palpation and diagnosis by the five colors, the presumptive content of the lost text he cited, thus connecting him back to the energetic tradition started by Jiudai Ji.[99] Chunyu Yi was renowned for his prognostic abilities, due no doubt to these techniques.

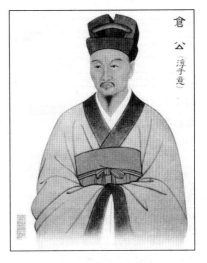

Figure 65: CHUNYU YI (216–155 B.C.)
The "father of case histories" who used his clinical records to defend himself against an accusation of malpractice.

Another Han dynasty physician, Guo Yu (first century A.D.), a disciple of Fu Weng, the Old Gentleman of the Fu river, who wrote a treatise on acupuncture and also developed his own method of pulse diagnosis, had his biography included in the *Annals of the Latter Han*. There he gives the traditional point of view in the ongoing controversy about how exacting a practitioner must be in locating the acupuncture points for treatment:

> "Even the slightest, hairline deviation, when inserting an acupuncture needle is an inexcusable professional blunder. The skillful practice of acupuncture depends upon perfect coordination of the mind and hands. It can be learned, but not described in words."[100]

Guo Yu's point of view is noteworthy because the fervor of his beliefs carries an implicit expression of the reliance traditionalists place on virtue (de), which is lost when acupuncture is separated from its traditional roots.[101]

The most astonishing physician of the Han dynasty was no doubt Hua Tuo (also known as Fu and Yuan Hua) (110–207 A.D.) who was memorialized in the *Annals of the Latter Han*, the *History of the Three Kingdoms*, and a popular novel, *The Romance of the Three Kingdoms*

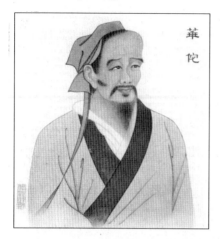

華
佗

Figure 66: HUA TUO (110–207 A.D.)
The "father of surgery" who operated using herbal anaesthesia, he
was also a brilliant acupuncturist,
using only one or two points
per treatment.

(Fig.66). While he contributed to practically every branch of medicine, his face and name are indelibly associated with acupuncture, appearing as the trademark of the first brand of acupuncture needles to be exported by China. In the practice of acupuncture he was noted for the use of only one or two points per treatment during which he would tell his patients what they should expect to feel; as soon as they reported these sensations the needles were withdrawn and the illnesses were subsequently cured.[102] The simplicity and power of his style of acupuncture set a standard aimed at by many subsequent practitioners, though largely ignored by others. In honor of his contributions to acupuncture, the series of Extraordinary acupuncture Points located one half inch lateral to the spine were named "Hua Tuo Jia Ji" Points,[103] and it is believed that he used these locations in preference to the more commonly used back Shu Points.[104] It is not as an acupuncturist, however, that Hua Tuo is most famous, but rather in his role as the "father of surgery." He discovered a method of herbal anaesthesia and performed numerous operations on every part of the body including the viscera and brain. In fact, it was his recommendation of brain surgery to Emperor Cao Cao

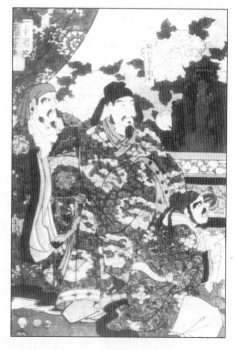

whose headaches he diagnosed as being due to a brain tumor, which cost this great physician his life. Unfortunately, Cao Cao suspected that the proposed operation was a clever attempt at assassination, and took his revenge by having Hua Tuo decapitated at the age of 97![105] One of Hua Tuo's more famous operations was his debridement of a poisoned-arrow wound in the arm of General Guan Yu, an immensely popular war hero who was subsequently deified. When Guan Yu was wounded in battle, Hua Tuo was called to operate and offered his anaesthetic potion. Guan Yu merely laughed and distracted himself with a game of "Go" while the surgery proceeded. This tableau has been a favorite subject of Oriental artists (Fig.67). Hua Tuo also originated several modalities of physical therapy including hydrotherapy and therapeutic exercises. The latter he developed into the game of the five animals patterned after the tiger, deer, bear, monkey and crane, which undoubtedly were originally correlated to the Five Elements but whose details have unfortunately been lost along with virtually all the rest of Hua Tuo's discoveries, including his herbal anaesthetic and a vermifuge for insects in the stomach (Fig.68). A book called the *Classic of the Central Viscera* has been attributed to him, but most commentators believe it to be the work of an unknown Daoist who used Hua's name for its prestige.[106]

Having touched on Hua Tuo's pharmaceutical contributions, it is appropriate to note that starting "in the Han dynasty, people became

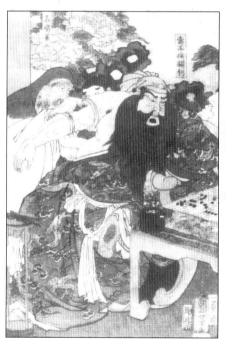
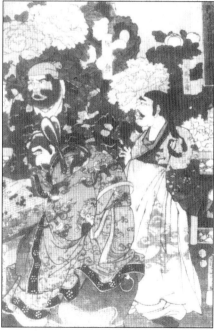

Figure 67: HUA TUO AND GUAN YU
Hua Tuo is seen operating on General Guan, debriding down to the bone, while the latter blithely ignores him in favor of the challenge of a game of "Go."

interested in herb medicine and lost their enthusiasm in acupuncture and moxibustion"[107]. One can only speculate on what factors were responsible for this change. The Han dynasty was a peculiar one, split in the middle by Wang Mang's usurpation of the throne, and philosophically it may similarly be broken into two parts: the former Han period (202 B.C.–9 A.D.) gave birth to the last of the great philosophical Daoist classics, the *Huai-Nan Zi* (c. 122 B.C.),[108] while the later Han period (25 A.D.–220 A.D.) saw the origin of religious Daoism based on two

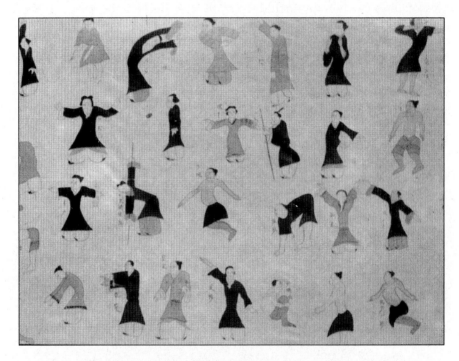

Figure 68: TAO YIN.
Various systems of therapeutic exercise have been incorporated into TOM throughout history. Hua Tuo developed the "game of the five animals" during the Han dynasty, and although his system has been lost, this chart illustrates another approach from the same era. It was recovered from the Han dynasty number three tomb at Mawangdui.

rebellious groups known as the "Way of Great Peace" or "Yellow-Turbans" on the one hand and the "Way of the Five Bushels of Rice" or followers of the Daoist "Pope" Zhang Dao-ling on the other[109] (Fig.69). As Daoism was the major philosophical and spiritual basis for traditional Oriental medicine, it is not unreasonable to suspect that as

Daoism changed, so would Oriental medicine. Practitioners of the healing arts at this time were called "fang shi" or masters of prescriptions, and it is in this category that one finds Hua Tuo. De Woskin traces the lineage from wu shi (shamans) to fang shi to dao shi (Daoist adepts).[110]

One of the main differences between philosophical and religious Daoism was in their attitude toward death. The philosophical school taught a spiritual path towards the loss of consciousness of self, and thereby a transcendence of death, while the religious approach was to banish death itself by reaching physical immortality. The former tried "by mystic insight to transcend man's limitations," while the latter tried "by magic and protoscience, not to change man's understanding of what life is, but to perpetuate and ameliorate precisely the life he knows."[111] Physical means of accomplishing this were prominent from the start, as Zhang Dao-ling, the founder of religious Daoism, was himself an alchemist.[112] In fact, the earliest alchemical treatise, *The Kinship of the Three* by Wei Po Yang was written in 142 A.D., during Zhang's lifetime.[113] Alchemy, as a method of achieving immortality, was based on the ingestion of natural substances including animal, vegetable and mineral products, which makes the alchemical tradition intimately connected with that of herbal medicine.

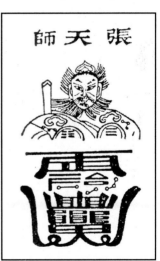

Several primitive works on herbal medicine dating from the Han dynasty have been discovered in recent years. *The Fifty-two Prescriptions* from Ma wang dui and the wooden tablets from Wu Wei in Gansu province both provide empirical formulae for prescribing herbs without discussing their theoretical basis.[114]

Traditionally, the origin of herbal medicine is attributed to the legendary Emperor Shen Nong, and while several ancient texts had mentioned individual herbs[115], the first book solely about herbs and their use which provided a theoretical underpinning was written by an unknown Han dynasty author who honorarily attributed it to Shen Nong. It was *Shen Nong's Materia Medica*, a work which listed 365 herbs in three classes, with a theory of prescriptive formulation and 170 diseases susceptible to herbal treatment. The original text was lost during the Tang dynasty.[116]

Figure 69:
ZHANG DAO-LING.
The originator of one sect of religious Daoism, Zhang was considered the Daoist Pope, and was famous for the use of charms and incantations to cure disease.

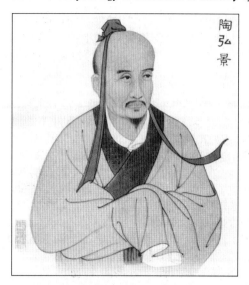

Figure 70: DAO HONG-JING (452–536 A.D.),
was a religious Daoist who salvaged and expanded the original herbal text known as *Shen Nong's Materia Medica.*

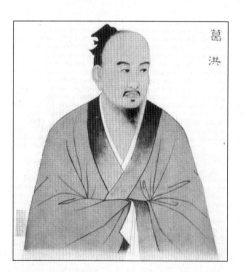

Figure 71: GE HONG (281–341 A.D.),
was a prolific writer on Daoist alchemy, more commonly known by his pseudonym Bao Pu Zi.

What we know of the original *Material Medica* is based on the work of a later Daoist alchemist, Dao Hong-jing (452-536 A.D.) who added 365 new herbs to the previous work and expanded the system of herbal classification[117] (Fig.70). The link I've proposed between herbalism and religious Daoism is supported by the inclusion of his work and other herbal texts in the *Dao Zang*, or Daoist Bible.[118] An earlier alchemist, Ge Hong (281-341 A.D.) whose works were also included in the *Dao Zang* under the pseudonym Bao Pu Zi,[119] explained the meaning of the three classes of herbs as being: Upper class: those which give immortality, middle class: those which prolong life and lower class: those which cure sickness (Fig.71). Ge Hong wrote prolifically, his works being even more extensive than those of the great historian Si Ma Qian. However he never undertook any alchemical experiments himself, due to the expense of the materials involved![120] While this revelation brings into question the value of his teachings, it may have allowed him to live out a normal life-span, in contrast to some of the royal recipients of alchemical elixirs who died of heavy metal poisoning.[121]

This brief synopsis of the origin of herbal medicine serves to introduce the works of the most influential physician of the Han dynasty, and possibly in the entire history of Chinese medicine, Zhang Zhong-jing. (c. 150–210 A.D.)[122] (Fig.72). While Zhang occasionally used acupuncture as an adjunctive therapy, he was principally an herbalist, but more than that, he elaborated the systematics of the clinical practice of herbal medicine in a manner that is still followed to this day. His books *Treatise on Cold-Induced Disorders* and *Essential Prescriptions of the Golden Chest*[123] along with the *Nei Jing* and *Nan Jing* are considered the canons of Oriental medicine.[124] Originally, his two works were published as one, *Treatise on Cold-Induced and Miscellaneous Diseases*, but as with the *Nei Jing*, no copies of the original work have survived. Although Zhang was familiar with the *Nei Jing* and *Nan Jing*, his work is a radical departure from them. He presents a schema for classifying cold-induced diseases in six stages, which borrows its terminology, but little else, from the *Nei Jing*. It is based on classifying symptoms and signs according to Yin/Yang theory, and uses a rudimentary form of the Eight Principles which form the basis of Traditional

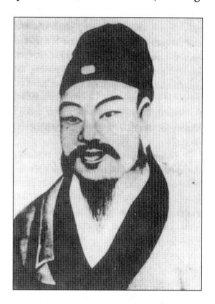

Figure 72: ZHANG ZHONG-JING
(c. 150–210 A.D.),
author of the *Shang Han Lun (Treatise on Cold-Induced Disorders)* which was the first clinical guide to the practice of Chinese herbal medicine, and is still revered today as the "Father of Prescriptions."

Chinese Medicine, or TCM.[125] Zhang introduced the etiological classification of illnesses as being due to endogenous, exogenous or miscellaneous causes, which is the root of the contemporary traditional theory of etiology developed approximately 1,000 years later in the Song dynasty.[126] The common theme throughout all of Zhang's work is the organization of his approach to illnesses around classifying them by the "differentiation of symptom-sign complexes," which allowed his work to be presented in the form of a clinical manual, the first of its kind, and earning it the sobriquet, "Father of Prescriptions."[127]

From what I have said, it is clear that Zhang took traditional Oriental medicine off in a new direction, and that the split in traditional acupuncture between the schools emphasizing the Five Elements (primarily outside the Peoples' Republic of China) and those emphasizing the Eight Principles (primarily within the PRC itself), which has become most pronounced in the twentieth century, cannot be reconciled without an understanding of the relationship of Zhang's work to the earlier works of traditional medicine. Zhang himself claimed to have studied books on herbs and the pulse in addition to the *Nei Jing* and *Nan Jing*.[128] In the Han dynasty, there were several dozens of medical treatises extant which were later lost[129] and I have already mentioned the nascent alchemical literature, all of which could have influenced Zhang's thinking. Many theories have been proposed to account for Zhang's tradition, but I think we are on the safest ground by sticking to that mentioned by Huang Fu Mi in the preface to his own book of 282 A.D., because it is the oldest medical text that has come down to us in its original form. In it, Huang states that the *Treatise on Cold-Induced Disorders* was based on the *Theory of Herbal Decoctions* attributed to Yi Yin, the prime minister of the ancient Yin (Shang) dynasty.[130] This theory has been the consensus belief of the Japanese who have tried to practice Zhang's herbology in its unadulterated form, and it links Zhang to an ancient branch of traditional Oriental medicine parallel to that of the *Nei Jing*.

This interpretation still leaves us with two unreconciled approaches to Oriental medicine, however the Japanese scholarship includes evidence that Zhang's work via Yi Yin was in turn ultimately based on the *Yi Jing*.[131] The implicit integration of Yin/Yang and 5 Element energetics, in the *Yi Jing* which was probably written shortly after the fall of the Shang dynasty, could thereby have served as the common source for later elaborations in both the *Nei Jing* and the *Treatise on Cold-Induced Disorders* (by way of the intermediary *Theory of Herbal Decoctions*). I have previously published a monograph which develops this hypothesis, showing that the six stages model of Zhang's *Treatise on Cold-Induced Disorders* is implicit in the Fu Xi circular order of the trigrams (which also appears in the *Nei Jing*) and that the Five Element model, more emphasized in the acupuncture tradition, is implicit in the Wen Wang order of the trigrams.[132] I believe this to be a credible solution to the dilemma of two competing traditions which ultimately only emphasized different aspects of the coherent energetic theories embodied in the *Yi Jing*.

The two prominent physicians of the subsequent Jin dynasty (265–420 A.D.) were each linked to Zhang Zhong-jing. Wang Shu-he salvaged Zhang's original one volume text and divided it into the two that are now extant (Fig.73). He is much more famous, however, for his own book, the *Classic of Pulses*, written in 280 A.D., which was the first comprehensive work on the subject. On the one hand, it clarifies the correspondences of Meridians and viscera to the 12 radial pulse positions as they were presented in the *Nan Jing*, and on the other hand it systematizes the different pulse qualities and divides them into 24 types giving in addition their diagnostic significance. Wang was thus clearly an expert in both the *Nei Jing* and *Treatise on Cold-Induced Disorders* traditions, and made no mention of any fundamental discrepancy between them, thus reassuring us in the hypothesis of a unitary conception. The *Classic of Pulses* was widely disseminated throughout the world, and even influenced Arabic medicine, showing up as the 24 pulses in Avicenna's *Medical Dictionary* in the eleventh century.[133]

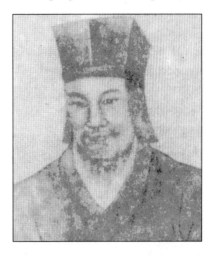

Figure 73: WANG SHU-HE (210–285 A.D.), author of the *Mai Jing (Classic of Pulses)*, a work whose influence extended even into Arabic medicine.

The other famous Jin physician, Huang Fu Mi has already been mentioned in regard to his contribution to the discussion of the origins of the *Treatise on Cold-Induced Disorders* (Fig.74). He is also much more famous for his own book, the *Systematic Classic of Acupuncture and Moxibustion* written in 282 A.D. This was the first book solely about acupuncture and moxibustion, and filled in many of the gaps in the earlier literature. It lists 349 acupuncture Points by Meridian and region, giving their names, locations, properties, indications and methods of treatment in terms of needle depth, duration of needling, and number of moxa cones to be applied.[134] In addition it introduces a new method, treating physiologically defined Points, the Xi or Accumulation Points,[135] for acute symptoms, something which had not been described in the *Nei Jing* or *Nan Jing*. This work became the basic text in the field not only in China but also in Japan and Korea,[136] and to reiterate, it is the oldest traditional medical text to have survived intact into the present. It is of interest to note that when Huang was about 40 years old which was near the beginning of his professional life, he suffered from a serious illness that has been variously reported as either a stroke[137] or a severe attack of rheumatism.[138] In any case, his subsequent career belies the frequently stated, but erroneous belief that an acupuncturist must be in excellent health in order to practice effectively. The opposite view is also supported by the career of Sun Si-Miao, the most famous physician of the Tang dynasty, who was likewise in poor health,

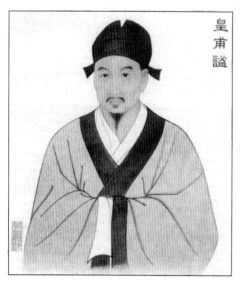

皇
甫
謐

**Figure 74: HUANG-FU MI
(215–286 A.D.),**
author of *Jia Yi Jing (Systematic Classic
of Acupuncture and Moxibustion)*, the
first book to provide a reasonably comprehensive presentation of the classical
acupuncture Points.

but who successfully treated himself[139] thereby violating yet another dogmatic proscription.[140] It is my own belief that actually, rather than subtracting from one's powers, the experience of illness in the physician himself and his attempts to grapple with it, strengthens him in his bond with his patients. After all, Oriental medicine is not so much based on intellectual knowing as it is on experiential being.

Returning to our history, we have covered developments through the Jin dynasty, i.e. 420 A.D. The next 700 years or so were mostly devoted to the elaboration of all the aspects of traditional Oriental medicine presented so far, particularly from the pedagogical point of view. Beginning with the Northern Wei dynasty, in 493 A.D. there was an Imperial Medical College under the Imperial Medical Service[141] devoted to the promulgation of Oriental medicine and divided into four departments which illustrates the components of traditional medicine at that time—internal and external medicine, acupuncture and moxibustion, massage, and demonology (i.e., shamanism).[142] About 495 A.D. the oldest extant book on external medicine appeared,[143] discussing surgery, trauma, skin diseases and antiseptic technique. Then in 610 A.D., in the Sui dynasty (581–618 A.D.) *Chao's Etiology*[144] provided the first comprehensive exposition of etiology and pathology, presenting over 1700 articles on disease symptomatology and its treatment, primarily by acupuncture (Fig.75). Chao Yuan-fang, the Taiyi or physician to the Emperor was in a unique position to achieve such a compilation. However, the most important advance in the field of acupuncture at this time was the appearance of teaching tools not based on discursive methodology—i.e., the development of meridian charts and statues.

It is not known exactly when the first charts were produced, although there is reason to believe they date back to the Han dynasty.[(145)] We do know that Sun Si-Miao (590–682 A.D.) in the Tang dynasty (618–906 A.D.) drew charts of the anterior, posterior and lateral views of the body, the same format in use today, and showed the Principal Meridians in five colors with the Extraordinary Meridians in a sixth color (Fig.76). Sun is also credited with the introduction of the system of proportional measurement, the "Chinese inch," which allows for accurate localization in spite of individual differences in size and shape.[(146)] The pinnacle of this development was the casting of two life-size bronze manikins by Wang Wei-i (Fig.77) in 1027 A.D., in the Song dynasty (960–1279 A.D.). These models had holes at the locations of the acupuncture Points, and were constructed in such a way that they could be covered with a thin layer of wax and then filled with water (Fig.78). Students were required to pierce the wax in the correct places, so as to allow the water to flow out.[(147)] In my visits to acupuncture schools in both the Orient and Occident, I have never seen such a device in use, but it appeals to my esthetic sense, and I hope it will someday be resurrected. I should point out however, that an influential Japanese tradition teaches that the Points are living phenomena which can actually change location with varying states of health, and thus must be individually located by using refined palpatory skills in each separate patient.

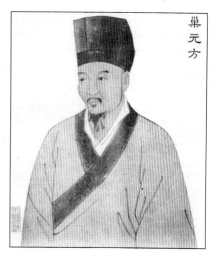

Figure 75: CHAO YUAN-FANG (550–630 A.D.) author of *Zhu Bing Yuan Hou Zhong Lun (Chao's Etiology)*, the first comprehensive work on etiology and pathology in Chinese medicine.

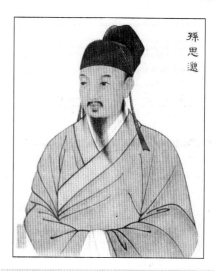

Figure 76: SUN SI-MIAO (590–682 A.D.) the most esteemed physician of the Tang dynasty, who contributed to nearly every branch of TOM including ethics, acupuncture, moxibustion, herbal medicine and demonology.

I have previously mentioned Sun Si-Miao in several contexts: ethics, self-treatment, charts and proportional measurement. In this I have only scratched the surface of his many contributions to Oriental medicine. Thus, it is curious that Sun was not at all favorable to

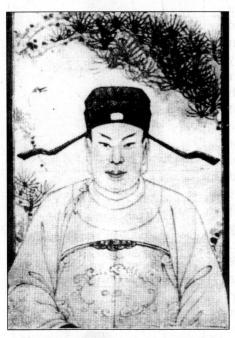

acupuncture in his early years, but concentrated his attention on herbal medicine and nutrition. His cautious attitude towards acupuncture reflected the recognition that it could do as much harm as good, a dilemma that has colored physicians' attitudes towards acupuncture down to the present day. In Sun's case, his caution caused him to adopt a critically observant approach and from this foundation, when he finally endorsed acupuncture, he was able to introduce and systematize many new concepts including the categories of "Forbidden Points," "Ah Shi" or "Ouch" Points, "Extraordinary Points," and Points for preventative scarring moxibustion, in addition to his charts and system of proportional measurement.[148]

Figure 77: WANG WEI-I,
a Song dynasty acupuncturist who supervised the casting of two life-size bronze manikins under imperial patronage.

Not all of the prominent physicians of the Tang dynasty were convinced, however, that acupuncture could be practiced with safety and efficacy. In particular, Wang Tao (675–755 A.D.), the most prolific medical writer of his day,[149] dealt with herbal medicine and moxibustion but not acupuncture, feeling that the latter was likely to injure a patient instead of saving him[150] (Fig.79). Wang did, however, institute a new tradition in Oriental medicine, by stating the sources for all of the prescription formulae he collected, a fashion which has regrettably not been universally followed.[151]

The confusion over the correct path for Oriental medicine was only exacerbated by the behavior of the Tang emperor, Yi Zong, who was furious when his daughter died of a febrile illness in spite of the best medical care available. In his bitterness, Yi Zong ordered the beheading of twenty of the leading Chinese physicians.[152]

Although Oriental medicine was beset with many challenges during the Tang dynasty, one of its greatest achievements was the publication of the revised edition of the *Nei Jing* by Wang Bing-ci in 762. As I have mentioned, Wang (c. 710–804 A.D.) is thought to have added at least seven chapters of his own (Chapters 66–71 and 74) to replace those already lost by his time,[153] and it is the nature of his innovative replacements that I would like to consider next. His "new" chapters deal with what Porkert has called "phase energetics," which literally translates from the Chinese as "five phases and six energies."[154] Because traditional acupuncture is based on the notion of the controlled manipulation of energy, the systematization of phase energetics was an important advance.[155] The origin of the concept of phase energetics is controversial, some authorities tracing this idea back to the Han dynasty while others place it as late as the Tang.[156] In either case, it is clear that it is not until after the Tang that the commentatory literature began to discuss phase energetics, and to describe concretely how to give acupuncture

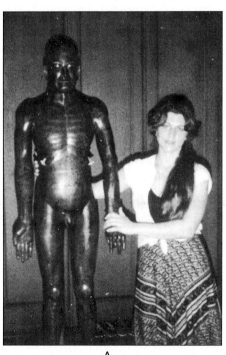
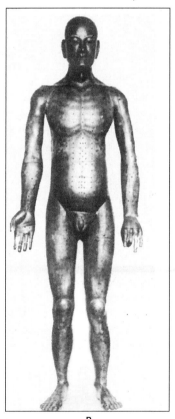

A   B

Figure 78: THE BRONZE MANIKIN.
This copy is in the National Museum in Tokyo, where it may be seen by special arrangement.

treatment with respect to the hour, day, month and season. Particular applications of phase energetics in acupuncture include the Law of Midday/Midnight, the Four-Needle Technique, and treatment by the

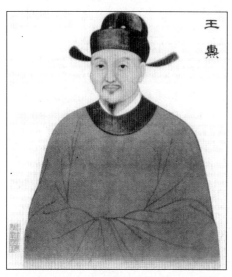

王
燾

Stems and Branches, all of which depend on a knowledge of the 66 Command Points on the 12 Principal Meridians. (More information on these technical terms can be found in the Appendix, but they can safely be skipped over by the lay reader without loosing the thread of this story.) The point I would like to emphasize is that the "five phases and six energies" involve a thorough integration of the twin theoretical bases of Five Elements and Yin/Yang doctrines and is fully in keeping with the prior developments in traditional acupuncture.

Figure 79: WANG TAO (675–755 A.D.) dissapproved of acupuncture as being too dangerous. He favored moxibustion and herbal medicine instead.

The interest in phase energetics developed side by side with a comprehensive re-evaluation of traditional metaphysical teachings in the Song dynasty, a movement known as Neo-Confucianism. This development was essentially an attempt to account for manifest reality on the basis of a more systematic description of the workings of the Dao. In Neo-Confucian terms, the Supreme Ultimate or Tai Ji is the state of unmanifest reality which (through the workings of the Dao) gives rise to all manifest phenomena through the interaction of primal substrate (Qi) and the principle (Li) which organizes it. The following Song philosophers were important in developing this theory: Zhou Dunyi (1071–1073), Zhang Zai (1020–1077), Cheng Hao (1032–1085), Cheng Yi (1033–1107) and Zhu Xi (1130–1200). The familiar symbol for the interaction of Yin and Yang, known as the Tai Ji image (Fig.80) is a product of this era, and has now become the universally recognized emblem of traditional Oriental thought.

During this same period, a Bureau for Re-editing Medical Books was established in 1057, which had the effect of consolidating an "orthodox" tradition. The earliest extant text on the history of Chinese medicine, *Yishou* was written somewhat thereafter by Zang Gao, in 1189, so much of what we know of the early history of Chinese medicine most likely has a Neo-Confucian bias. In any case, the introduction of phase energetics together with the other Neo-Confucian metaphysical speculations, seems to have sparked a renewed interest in theorization in Oriental medicine in general, which led to major developments in herbal medicine as well, especially starting in the Jin (1115–1234 A.D.) and Yuan (1260–1368 A.D.) dynasties. The other springboard for these new theories was the clarification of traditional etiology by Chen Yen in 1174 A.D., when he elaborated on the classification of etiological factors into the three categories of exogenous, endogenous and miscellaneous.[157] These developments led to the "Four Great Schools" of the Jin and Yuan dynasties, whose teachings

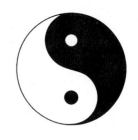

Figure 80:
THE TAI JI IMAGE
univerally recognized as a symbol of Yin and Yang, first became popular in the Song Dynasty.

became the most powerful orthodox tradition in China, becoming incorporated into TCM, but were not as universally accepted in Japan, which, after a preliminary trial of Jin-Yuan style medicine, subsequently harkened back to the *Treatise on Cold-Induced Disorders* for its style of Oriental herbal medicine and to the *Nei Jing* and especially the *Nan Jing* for its style of traditional acupuncture.

The "cooling" school of Liu Wan-su[158] (1120–1200 A.D.) was the first of the "Four Great Schools"[159] (Fig.81). Based on a discussion of phase energetics, Liu developed the idea that exogenous pathogens (the "six energies") universally provoked heat and inflammation in the body. Therefore, he recommended treatment of all such conditions with cold and cool drugs, but he also recommended acupuncture and incantations as adjunctive treatment. His herbal teachings are widely known, whereas his thoughts about acupuncture are

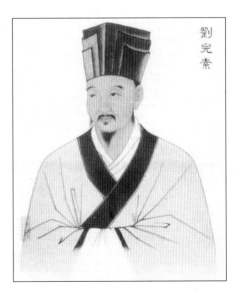

Figure 81: LIU WAN-SU
(1120–1200 A.D.),
founder of the "cooling" school of thought.

not, and although he wrote three books on the *Su Wen* his methods of acupuncture are said to have been maintained only by a few expatriates who continued his oral tradition on China's offshore islands.[160]

In contrast, Li Dong-yuan (1180–1251 A.D., also known variously as Li Gao or "the old gentleman of the Eastern wall")[161] focused his attention on the endogenous and miscellaneous causes of disease, and concluded that these all act to disrupt the functioning of the Stomach and Spleen in their nutritional role of supporting the body's "original energy"[162] (Fig.82). His publication of these ideas in 1249 A.D. lead to the "strengthening the Earth" school which recommended strengthening the Stomach and Spleen with tonics as the basic approach to all treatment.[163] Like Liu Wan-su, some of his work is much less well known (perhaps because it is outside the usual domain of TCM), and includes the use of psychosomatic treatments for dealing with cases of excessive joy, anger, sadness, grief, fear and apprehension.[164]

Zhang Cong-zheng[165] (1156 –1228 A.D.) was a military physician who disagreed with the theories of both Liu and Li, and instead proposed that all illnesses were basically due to excessive pathogenic factors in the climate or diet which needed to be expelled from the body (Fig.83). Thus, he developed the "purgative" school which favored diaphoretics, emetics and purgatives over tonics, and his style of acupuncture emphasized the use of the bleeding needle.[166]

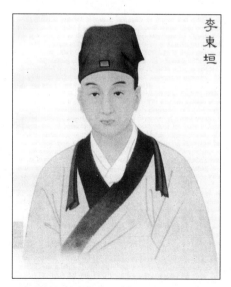

Figure 82: Li Dong-yuan (1180–1251 A.D.), founder of the "strengthening the Earth" school of thought.

Finally, Zhu Zhen-heng (1281 –1358 A.D., also known as Master Danxi)[167] developed a fourth universal explanation for disease: that internal deficiency resulting from overindulgence was the root cause, and he taught that all illnesses must therefore be treated with tonics (Fig.84). He focussed on the difference between "princely" and "ministerial" types of fire,[168] and explained that excessive activity of the latter has the effect of weakening Yin. Based on this pathological model, in 1347 A.D. he published the doctrine that it was always Yin which became Deficient, while Yang tended to Excess, and his recommendations led to the "nourishing the Yin" school.[169] He also contributed to the development of the doctrine initiated by Zhang Yuan-su (c. 1186) that herbs work by "entering" different Meridians in the body,[170] thereby trying to re-establish a connection between acupuncture and herbal medicine, which had become weakened by the new herbalist theories of the Four Schools. Earlier authors had proposed conflicting schemes for which herbs entered which Meridians, but Zhu added the notion that because individual herbs can have several different flavors in combination, each one could enter several different Meridians, a resolution which has continued to this day to be the dominant interpretation. Zhu is also associated with another method or school called the "living noose" which referred to a type of "word therapy" wherein the practitioner embodied different emotions in an attempt to induce different affective reactions in patients[171]—a technique that today is allocated at least as much clinical practice time as is pulse diagnosis in the Leamington Acupuncture schools, while being virtually unknown in those of TCM or other traditions.

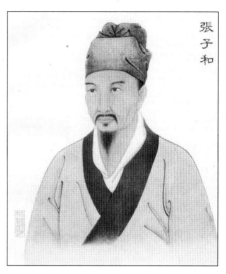

Figure 83: ZHANG CONG-ZHENG
(1156–1228 A.D.)
founder of the "purgative" school of thought.

While these four schools were primarily concerned with herbal medicine, they have broader implications for all of Oriental medicine, which they have influenced. Each school took some aspect of etiology and tried to formulate a system of therapeutics appropriate to deal with the chosen causative factor. The danger of such approaches is that they necessarily ignore essential parts of Oriental medicine by seeing all ill-ness from the viewpoint of a specific etiological category. The strength of Oriental medicine, on the other hand, has always rested on its holis-tic conceptualization and willingness to treat each individual without any preconceptions as to why they might be sick. We can see this same tendency towards ideological (and etiological) narrowing in the surviv-ing contemporary styles of traditional acupuncture, all of which suffer to the degree that they exclude parts of the totality of TOM, including, but not limited to: the relative importance of Yin/Yang versus Five Element doctrines, endogenous (psychological) versus exogenous (somatic) etiological factors, and even the role of the Spirit and the pos-sibility of demonic possession.

I am not the first author to comment on the fragmentation of Oriental medicine into opposing schools of herbalism and acupuncture. Cheng et. al.[172] noted this separation as occurring in the Yuan dynasty and attributed it to a conflict between theoreticians (the herbalists) on

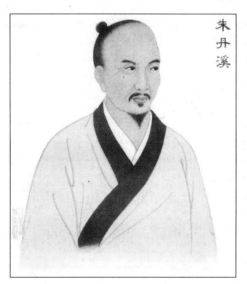

the one hand and practitioners (the acupuncturists) on the other. Needham takes the opposite view, that the establishment of phase energetics in acupuncture represented the unfortunate triumph of abstract theory over clinical practice.[173] Being neither a practitioner, nor even a proponent of traditional acupuncture, his value judgments in this regard should be taken weighed accordingly. It was, in fact, Dou Han-qing's (1195–1280)[174] systematic application of phase energetics to acupuncture around 1241 A.D.[175] that allowed for the development of more reliable protocols for specific energetic interventions in acupuncture therapy. These included the use of the Command or Crossing Points of the Eight Extraordi-

Figure 84: Zhu Zhen-heng (1281–1358 A.D.), founder of the "nourishing the Yin" school of thought.

nary Meridians, which he was the first to describe.[176] His book, *Zhenjing Zhinan* was reprinted with several others including He Ruoya's *Ziwuliuzhu Zhenjing* in a 1331 compendium by his son Dou Guifang (also known as Tu Shih-ching) that established the role of the five Shu Points (also known as Five Element or Antique Points) in phase energetic therapy. Dou Han-qing was also the originator of many of the poetic names for the more complex needle techniques such as, "Setting the Mountain on Fire" for simultaneous tonification and heating, and "Making Cool like a Clear Sky" for simultaneous dispersion and cooling.[177] Another development of phase energetics, the notion of open and closed times for acupuncture Points and Meridians, was due to the Yuan dynasty physician Hua Shou (1304–1386) who was also the first author to classify the Governing and Conception Vessels with the twelve Principal Meridians, to make up the fourteen Meridians that have their own Points.[178]

Moving on to the Ming dynasty (1368–1644) Gao Wu,[179] adapting ideas proposed by Xu Feng [180] (*Zhen Jiu Da Quan*, 1439), published *Zhen Jiu Ju Ying* in 1529, introducing the concept of Tonification and Sedation Points as special cases of the 66 Command Points, thus allowing for more systematic and practical use of Five Element theory in acupuncture treatment.[181] He also systematized the needle techniques for tonification and dispersion by both twisting and rotating and by lifting and thrusting.[182] Li Yan, also known as Li Zhai-jian, further developed the rules for tonification and dispersion in *Yi Xue Ru Men* or *The Basics of Medical Studies* (1575) which specified the needle methods according to male-female, left-right, Yang-Yin and inhale-exhale. This work had a marked influence on the development of traditional acupuncture in the West as we will see in Chapter Five.[183] In 1624 A.D., Zhang Jie-bin[184] wrote the *Classic of Categories* which systematized the disparate information in the ancient classics, and also introduced the idea of differentiating the "six changes," a primitive form of what later developed into the differentiation by the Eight Principles, which is the diagnostic rubric of TCM[185] (Fig.85). Zhang also introduced the original song of ten questions which embodies the standard form of interrogative investigation in TCM.

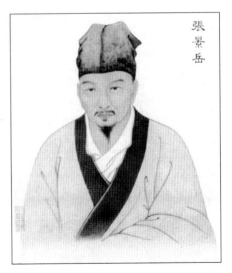

Finally, he is also remembered as the founder of the school of Yang tonification.[186] Perhaps the height of acupunctural scholarship was reached by Yang Ji-zhou (1522–1620 A.D.)(Fig.86), whose *Great Compendium of Acupuncture and Moxibustion,* published in 1601 A.D., summarized all the prior discoveries and teachings.[187]

Unfortunately, this pinnacle of traditional acupuncture was not long maintained. During the Ming dynasty, the split between the scholar physicians and the familial practitioners became more entrenched. In fact, one of the latter, Zhao Xue-min[188] (c.1730 –1805 A.D.) became quite famous although he used an approach that was not based on the classical teachings of either Yin/Yang or

Figure 85: ZHANG JIE-BIN (1563–1640 A.D.), founder of the "Yang tonification" school of thought.

Five Element theory, but rather on the idea that herbs have their effects based on four properties: ascending nature, descending nature, inter-

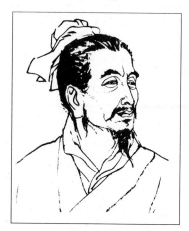

Figure 86: YANG JI-ZHOU
(1522–1620 A.D.),
author of the *Great Compendium
of Acupuncture and Moxibustion,*
an epochal work which contains
the seeds of the various styles of
traditional acupuncture as practiced in the twentieth century, to
be discussed in Chapter Five.

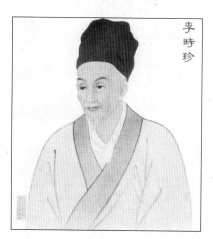

Figure 87: LI SHI-ZHEN
(1518–1593 A.D.)
author of the *Ben Cao Gang Mu
(Great Pharmacopaea)* whose
influence reached to both
Linnaeus and Darwin.

rupters of pathological processes and
repellers of exogenous pathogenic factors. His ideas have nevertheless been
subsequently incorporated into traditional herbal theory.[189]

As time went on, more and more
emphasis was placed on herbal medicine. This must have been due, at
least partially, to the monumental
work of China's greatest naturalist, Li
Shi-zhen (1518–1593 A.D.)[190] who
after 40 years of research published
the *Great Pharmacopaea* in 1578 A.D.,
listing over 1800 herbs and 1,000 prescriptions, a work which has had
world-wide impact and is felt to have
influenced both Linnaeus and
Darwin[191] (Fig.87). Li was also interested in acupuncture, however, and
wrote a book on the Eight Extraordinary
Meridians as well as one on pulse
diagnosis in which he described the
27 classical pulse qualities.[192]

The tide continued to turn more
toward herbal medicine and away
from acupuncture. In 1532 A.D.,
Wang Ji (1463–1539 A.D.)[193] published a book called *Questions and
Answers on Acupuncture* in which he
stated, "Acupuncture can cure diseases of abundance, but not those of
deficiency" and he strongly criticized
the mechanical application of phase
energetics to acupuncture, having
himself suffered from "incompetent
treatment by those who pretended to
know, while not knowing at all."[194]
Also, several new ideas were hotly
debated during the Ming dynasty. The
importance of the Fire of the Vital
Gate or "Ming Men" and its differentiation from the Right Kidney as it
was described in the *Nan Jing* was discussed by Zhao Xian-ke[195] (c. 1687

A.D.) who stressed that the Kidney as an embodiment of the Element Water, controls the Fire of the Vital Gate.[196] Both Wang and Zhao made memorable contributions to the practice of herbal medicine, the former popularizing the prescriptions known as Si Jun Zi Tang and Ba Zhen Tang, while the latter did the same for both Ba Wei and Liu Wei Di Huang Tang, all famous prescriptions in common use today in TCM.[197] Around the same time, Li Zhong-zi[198] (died 1655 A.D.) developed the idea that the Kidney and the Spleen were the roots of the inherited and the acquired constitutions, respectively,[199] a doctrine which accounts for the subsequent focus of TCM on these two Organs in almost every illness. This approach was a natural outgrowth of the synthesis of the various theories I mentioned as having been introduced in the Jin and Yuan dynasties.

Towards he end of the Ming dynasty, an outbreak of the plague decimated the provinces of Hebei, Shandong, Jiangsu and Zhejiang in 1641. Based on his experiences in treating its victims, the herbalist Wu You-xing[200] published a surprisingly "Western" treatise, the *Theory of Epidemics* in 1642 A.D., wherein he distinguished epidemics from ordinary infectious diseases and claimed they were due to disease substances or pestilential energy (li qi) which enter their victims through bodily orifices—nose, mouth, pores, etc. (Fig.88). It is interesting to note that the first European book on acupuncture was published only a few years later (1658 A.D.),[201] both works being harbingers of the cross-fertilization of Eastern and Western medical thought. Ironically, the causative bacillus of plague was actually discovered in Hong Kong, by Alexander Yersin in 1894.[202]

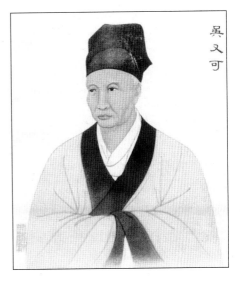

Figure 88: WU YOU-XING
(1582–1652 A.D.),
an herbalist whose theory of pestilential energy paralleled the Western concept of infectious diseases.

The last Chinese dynasty, the Qing, began in 1644 and lasted until 1911. The most significant developments in traditional medicine it produced were several herbal theories on how to treat illnesses due to exogenous heat (wen bing): The first was the theory of the Four Divisions[203] developed by Ye Tian-shi[204] in 1746 (Fig.89). An alternative approach based on the theory of the Three

Heaters was developed by Wu Ju-tong[205] in 1798, and both of these theories became part of the orthodox teachings of TCM. While herbal medicine continued to experience some growth, traditional acupuncture all but died out. What remained of traditional acupuncture was a modern revision in which diagnoses were fomulated according to the system being developed for herbal medicine (which I am about to describe) for which matching acupuncture prescriptions were devised in which the Points were described as carrying out the functions formerly ascribed only to the individual herbs comprising each herbal prescription. For example, some Points were said to transform dampness, other Points to regulate the Blood, and still others to relieve the Exterior, etc. This development has been referred to as "the herbalization of acupuncture," a characterization first mentioned by Kaptchuk, and popularized by Flaws.[206] There were three refinements in the art of diagnosis during the Qing dynasty which paved the way for this evolution, each of which was ideally suited to the philosophy of the dialectical materialists who later formulated the specifics of TCM. The first and most significant factor was the formalization of the differentiation of syndromes according to the Eight Principles[207] by Cheng Zhong-ling (c. 1732, also known as Cheng Guo-peng), which as I have mentioned, has become emblematic of TCM[208] as has the Five Elements become emblematic of LA. Combined with the Eight Principles, was the determination of the "visceral system manifestation type,"[209] otherwise known as the syndromes of the Zang/Fu, or Organs. Sivin describes this as a "recent system of analysis which in effect leads the medical student from a list of symptoms, without further exercise of judgement, to a specific manifestation type." He points out that while the origins of this methodology go back to the "Classic of the Central Viscera" attributed to Hua Tuo (but more probably written in the Northern Song dynasty) it has only become highly ramified and widely used in the last generation. The third facet of this diagnostic approach was the systematization

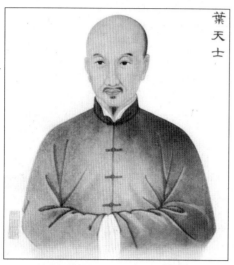

葉天士

Figure 89: YE TIAN-SHI (1667–1746 A.D.), developed the theory of the Four Divisions for combatting Heat diseases (wen bing).

and more generalized use of tongue diagnosis starting late in the nineteenth century, as exemplified in Zhou Xue-hai's *Simplified Study of External Diagnosis* written in 1894.[210] Although these three diagnostic methods were evolving during the Qing dynasty, (and later became pillars of the resurrected TCM) acupuncture itself was beginning a period of roughly two hundred years of virtual eclipse in China. Before looking at the reasons for this however, I would like to point out that the traditional forms of acupuncture which had been spreading out from China across the Orient, for the most part did not incorporate these most recent developments. Thus traditional acupuncturists in Japan for instance, usually have no familiarity with either tongue diagnosis, Zang/Fu syndromes, or the Eight Principles, and as a result, have been at a severe disadvantage in achieving licensure in those Western jurisdictions which use examinations largely based on the TCM approach to acupuncture.

As for the decline of acupuncture during the Qing dynasty, Needham cites a 1757 Chinese publication which speaks of acupuncture as a "lost art, for there were then left very few experts in it, and young physicians were at a loss to find teachers who could instruct them in it."[211] Why this happened is open to speculation. Lok Yee-Kung, a master practitioner who was personally trained by a member of the staff of astronomy under the last Qing Empress, relates that the rulers of the Qing dynasty (Manchus who were seen as occupying invaders by most of the Chinese) were afraid of the acupuncturists, because they thought the acupuncturists would murder them with their needles (Fig.90). Therefore, the royal family ordered acupuncture not to be used.[212] Needham cites the Confucian proscription against damaging or even exposing the body,[213] however, this explanation begs the question of why the decline of acupuncture occurred as late as the Qing dynasty. I prefer to think that the most important factor was the evolution of Oriental medical thought itself, which began to swing towards a greater interest in herbal medicine as early as the Han dynasty with the movement from philosophical to religious Daoism and its attendant alchemical teachings. The search was on for a corporeal "immortality" which demanded a pharmaceutical as opposed to an energetic methodology. Also, we should not underestimate the effect of the exposure of traditional China to western beliefs and practices, espe-

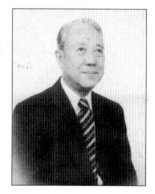

Figure 90:

LOK YEE-KUNG

a master acupuncturist trained by the royal astronomy staff under the last Qing Empress, now living in Las Vegas.

cially following China's defeat by the Western imperialist powers in the two Opium Wars in the mid 1800's. Western medicine spread rapidly once it was introduced into China, and all but eclipsed the indigenous health-care system. The Kang Xi emperor himself was successfully treated for a feverish illness with cinchona (Peruvian bark) supplied by a Jesuit missionary, de Fontaney,[214] culminating many years of Jesuit influence in the imperial court begun by Matteo Ricci in 1601. Finally, in 1822, the Imperial Government of Emperor Dao Guang issued a decree banning the teaching of acupuncture in the Imperial Medical College[215] and subsequently even the practice of acupuncture itself was banned.[216] Eventually, all of traditional medicine fell into disrepute as Western medicine became more widespread. There was an attempt to salvage Chinese medicine by combining it with Western medicine which produced the "School of Sino-Western Convergence and Intercourse" under the leadership of Tang Zong-hai (1846–1897), and a similar strategy was adopted by the leadership of the Taiping rebellion but neither achieved lasting success, although they undoubtedly influenced the form in which TCM re-emerged in the twentieth century. Chen Guo-fu, founder of the Institute for National Medicine, tried to explain the traditional medical theories of Yin/Yang and the Five Elements as no more than symbolic terminology for natural physiological processes, but as his critics pointed out, "if you replace the old medical ideas with universal scientific principles, why call it 'Chinese Medicine'?"[217] With the fall of the Chinese empire and its replacement by a republic, the minister of education under the Guo-min-dang was quoted in 1914 as saying, "I have decided to abolish Chinese medicine and to use no more Chinese remedies as well,"[218] a threat which was enacted into law in 1929.[219] With the subsequent communist revolution, there was no immediate change in attitude. As late as 1941, a prominent Marxist, T'an Chuang, could still call Chinese medicine, the "collected garbage of several thousand years."[220] However, the realities of the health needs of the Chinese people dictated that traditional medicine be allowed a place, and as early as 1928, Mao Ze-dong had advocated the use of "both Chinese and Western treatment,"[221] the blending of which was established as a goal by the National Conference on Health in Beijing in 1950. It was only in 1958, based on the prestige associated with the development of acupuncture "anesthesia," a feat which finally impressed even the Western world, that Mao made his famous remark, "Chinese medicine is a great treasure house! We must make all efforts to uncover it and raise its' standards."[222] This was at the beginning of the "Great Leap Forward" and a similar burst of publicity accompanied the introduction of the "Barefoot Doctors," who used techniques from both Chinese and Western medicine for emergency care, starting in 1966 with the "Great Proletarian Cultural Revolution."

Traditional acupuncture, having been "kept in the dark for hundreds of years" in China, was thus brought back into the light as TCM by a government that required all aspects of society to conform to the ideology of dialectical materialism. It is impossible to give a precise date for the origin of TCM,[223] but it should be understood that this approach is a modern development. Unschuld states that "earlier this century, the fiction of a so-called chung-i (Chinese medicine) was created—a conceptual system artificially extracted out of the wealth of tradition and presented in such a way that it appears to resemble Western medicine as a homogeneous system of ideas and practices."[224] Sivin concurs in noting that chung-i, officially translated as "Traditional Chinese Medicine," should be distinguished from the ideas and methods which have not survived modern reinterpretation, which he calls "classical medicine." He locates the separation of TCM and classical medicine as occurring "somewhat after 1900."[225] There has not been much material published, at least in English, which would document how TCM was thus created,[226] but the following observations should serve as a rough outline.

Two institutions seems to have exercised predominant control over this process: The Experimental Institute of Acupuncture and Moxibustion Therapy set up in 1951 under the Ministry of Public Health, and the Institute of Acupuncture and Moxibustion set up in 1955 under the Academy of Traditional Chinese Medicine.[227] The former Institute, under the directorship of Mme. Zhu Lian (1910–1978) (Fig.91A) emphasized the integration of Western medical concepts into TCM as seen in Figure 91B from her 1955 publication *New Study of Acupuncture and Moxibustion*. This book presents the acupuncture Points according to bodily regions, disregarding Meridian theory almost entirely. Under her guidance, electrical stimulation of acupuncture points, or electroacupuncture, was intensively studied and subsequently incorporated into the clinical methods of TCM. The second Institute, under the leadership of Cheng Dan-an (1899–1957) (Fig.92), the head of the TCM school of Jiangsu Province, probably played a greater role in codifying TCM theory. Flaws has this to say about his work: "Cheng Dan-an was in the early forefront of re-establishing acupuncture in China as a credible therapy. He created for himself and others a practical style suitable for mass instruction in Western style colleges to students influenced by Western educational methods. However, Cheng Dan-an himself organized and rationalized his acupuncture protocols strictly according to traditional Chinese medical theory and terminology. He did not admix his presentation with borrowings from Western medicine."[228] It should be kept in mind, however, that Cheng had also studied Western medicine, and was undoubtedly influenced by it. Kaptchuk has cited Cheng Dan-an as the source for the styles of treat-

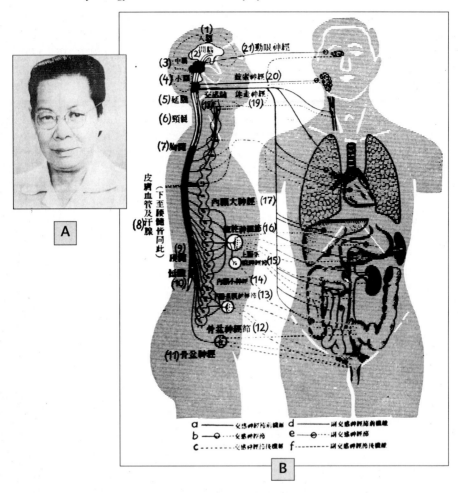

Figure 91: (A) ZHU LIAN (1910–1978),
director of the Experimental Institute of Acupuncture and Moxibustion
Therapy. (B) The Autonomic Nervous System, an illustration in Mme. Zhu's
New Study of Acupuncture and Moxibustion, which indicates her emphasis
on Western medical concepts.

ment now being used in TCM, which Cheng had been developing and
teaching since the 1930's.[229] Dr. Cheng was himself traditionally
trained, having studied under Chiu Chien-chuang and came from a
family of traditional medical practitioners, but was unusual in that he
had also studied in Japan and translated Japanese works on acupuncture
into Chinese.[230] It was after this experience that he founded one of the
first modern schools of acupuncture and moxibustion at Chengdu.[231]
Mme. Zhu on the other hand was obviously more deeply influenced by

her Western medical training.[232] Her work was important however, in that she had a significant international impact. She taught a seminal group of Russian doctors from 1956 to 1957 at her Institute in Beijing, and her book was reportedly used as a core teaching text in Vietnam.[233]

In 1955, both Zhu and Cheng published books under their own names, but more importantly in that year not only was the Academy of TCM established, but by then so were four of the five main colleges of TCM which were charged with developing a "modern curriculum" out of which the original textbooks of TCM were created.[234] According to Kaptchuk, it was during the 1950's that the Chinese medical schools developed the rationalizations of Acupoint functions which allowed for a fully herbalized approach to acupuncture.[235] Perhaps the clearest example of "herbalized acupuncture" was the work of Wang Le-ting (b. 1894) who compiled acupuncture formulae to specifically duplicate the effects of well-known herbal prescriptions, such as the widely used formula Shi Quan Da Bu Tang.[236] This prescription has ten herbal ingredients which are matched in a one to one correspondence by ten Acupoints having the same functions according to Wang, whose teachings were published in Beijing in 1984. A rationale for consciously "herbalizing" acupuncture has also been given by Peng Jingshan who wrote, "Herbal prescriptions are made according to the seven prescription and ten pharmaceutical forms, and this may be similarly applied to acupuncture, by simply changing herb names to acupuncture point names."[237]

It would be inaccurate however, to portray TCM as a rigid, unchanging discipline. Actually, depending on the political climate at the time, TCM has encompassed a wide variety of approaches—the one area it has never accommodated being the more mystical, spiritual and shamanistic practices; however, even that may be changing now with the recent interest in the medical uses of both external and internal Qi Gong. These practies are inextricably connected to meditation and other "spiritual" methods, and as yet have no experimentally verifiable material basis. More typical developments within TCM have included such diverse practices as acupuncture analgesia (first described as suitable for surgery in 1958)[238] and the injection of medications (both Western pharmaceuticals and Chinese herbs) into acupoints in attenuated dosages. The current Chinese approach to

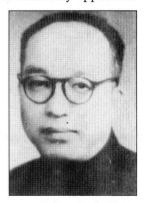

Figure 92: CHENG DAN-AN (1899 - 1957) director of the Institute of Acupuncture and Moxibustion, who perhaps played the leading role in codifying TCM theory and practice.

the development of TCM was made explicit in 1980–1981 as the "Three Roads" policy under which Western medicine, TCM and the integrated use of both together are all considered valuable and valid methods of health care, which should be allowed to freely develop according to their own inner logic.[239] Before finishing this presentation on the history of TCM, I would like to mention briefly its most materialist phase during the Cultural Revolution, when there was an attempt to expunge everything that could not be scientifically verified. During this time, "New Acupuncture" was developed in which only the Points were retained, the Meridians being dismissed as outmoded superstitution.[240]

I wanted to include the development of "New Acupuncture" in China because it paralleled earlier developments in Japan where the government in 1918, favoring the Western scientific outlook, compiled a list of "revised acupuncture points," which became the standard for licensure. The revised acupuncture points bore no resemblance to the traditional Meridians and Points, but were arbitrarily arranged according to a grid system superimposed over the surface of the body.[241] Naturally, this governmental decision provoked a reaction on the part of the proponents of traditional medicine, who in Japan had always been interested not only in the Chinese medical teachings, but also in their own spiritual tradition of Shinto, which as I have indicated was an early derivative of the form of shamanism that originally inspired the development of acupuncture in China and Korea. It is beyond the scope of this book to recount in detail the history of the development of acupuncture in Japan and the other countries of the Orient, or the struggles that were fought to preserve the purity of TOM, although I will have occasion to refer to it again. Suffice it to say that fortunately, classical TOM began to spread from China around the world at least as early as the Tang dynasty when it was transmitted to Japan, Korea and Vietnam.[242] Each of these countries developed its own style of acupuncture and Oriental medicine, and together with Taiwan and Hong Kong, preserved the parts of traditional acupuncture which later became unfashionable in China. Eventually, acupuncture spread to the West and today it is practiced, in one form or another, almost everywhere in the world. The final chapter presents my own attempts to recreate its journey to the West.

5

History as Mystery: Traditional Acupuncture's Journey to the West

While the preceeding chapters have presented the history of acupuncture from a chronological standpoint, the present chapter will take a different tack. As I have indicated, it is not my intention to describe the development of all the various traditions of acupuncture to be found in the West, but rather to focus on one of them, LA, and to report the findings I have personally uncovered in digging for its roots on and off over the last twenty years.

Let me begin by pointing out that regardless of how it may be commonly portrayed, LA is essentially a syncretic style of acupuncture, meaning that it combines methods and ideas from a number of different sources. I first realized the truth of this characterization in contemplating the integration of homeopathy into the syllabus of the Leamington College. Homeopathy is a non-conventional Western approach to medicine first developed in Germany in the nineteenth century, and as such could not have been part of any of the "classical" approaches to acupuncture or Oriental medicine. In fact, I do not know of any Oriental works that combine acupuncture and homeopathy, although as we shall see, there is a substantial precedent for such a combination in the West. I point this out because Worsley himself often says that what he teaches is the "traditional" or "classical" style of acupuncture transmitted to him via oral tradition by his teachers, and that they told him such teachings were handed down to them in this way from ancient times. This depiction of the purity of the classical teachings of LA must be taken with a grain of salt, for Worsley himself has also stated that he has personally tried every form of acupuncture currently being taught, including even the most clearly non-traditional method of electroacupuncture, and that he has formulated the syllabus of LA to include only what he has experienced as effective in promoting health of the Body, Mind and Spirit as a whole. This comment was made in the context of explaining why his students didn't need to repeat all the experiments and blind-alleys he went down in his own development. Such an admission clearly supports the hypothesis of LA as a syncretic approach.[243]

By now, the reader should have at least a basic understanding of the major differences between what I have been calling TCM and LA. Official TCM textbooks were first written in the 1950's—while the first comprehensive textbook of LA, on the other hand, has yet to be written![244] I point this out for the following reason: Worsley, as I just said, claimed that LA was received by him as an oral tradition, and as such he has continued to transmit it to his students. If, however, we are to embark on a search for its roots, we must know what methods and doctrines LA uniquely includes, so as to identify any precedents. Lacking a text which could serve such a purpose, I have compiled the following list, which is not meant to be either exhaustive or officially approved; it is merely my own set of observations and I have keyed it to the theory of the Circle presented in Chapters One and Two.

ATTRIBUTES OF LA

1) BASIC PRINCIPLES: The universe (manifestation of the Dao) follows Natural Laws. Only by recognizing these Laws of Nature, and by following them in our practice of acupuncture can we treat safely and effectively. The most important of these Laws in LA is the Law of the Five Elements, along with its corollaries: the Law of Mother-Son and the Creative (Sheng) and Control (Ke) cycles. The Law of Yin and Yang is given less emphasis, but actually takes priority over the Law of Five Elements if it has been violated seriously enough to create a Husband/Wife imbalance (see number 5 below). The original unity of the Dao is reflected in the unity of Body, Mind and Spirit which can never be separated, although they represent sequentially deeper levels of human existence. The deeper the level of imbalance, the more serious the illness.

2) VITAL FUNCTIONS: The human organism is governed by twelve Officials who are responsible for maintaining and developing all aspects of our lives in health and in illness. Each of these Officials also exists on the levels of Body, Mind and Spirit. As long as the twelve Officials are allowed to function according to the Natural Laws, they will stay in balance with each other and we as a result will stay healthy. Only when one or more of the Officials is malfunctioning will we become susceptible to illness.

3) VITAL STRUCTURE: Each of the twelve Officials has a pathway called a Meridian, where its vital energy (Qi) flows. The Officials are linked directly to the internal branch of their related Meridians, while the external or surface branch is that portion of the Meridian along which are located the acupuncture Points. Treatment here can help restore normal functioning to Officials that have become imbalanced.

Qi flows in a continuous cycle along these Meridians in a sequence that follows the Roman Numerals from I to XII, starting with the Heart, each Meridian experiencing a crest or waxing of its flow for two hours and a trough or waning of its flow for two hours every twenty-four hours. This cycle, reflecting the tides in the surface branches of the Meridians, is called the Wei or Protective cycle (as opposed to the deeper cycle of Qi flow according to the Five Elements) and the correlated two hourly peak for each Meridian is called the Law of Midday–Midnight. Each acupuncture Point has not only a traditional location (which may vary slightly in LA from the locations adopted in TCM) but also a traditional name which was chosen in antiquity to represent its therapeutic potential when stimulated in the appropriate circumstances. This energetic iconography is referred to in LA as the "Spirit of the Point." In regard to the Eight Extraordinary Meridians and the other so-called "Secondary Meridians" such as Divergent, Tendinomuscular and Longitudinal Connecting Meridians, in LA only the Governing and Conception Vessels, which have their own Points are included. The use of the other Extraordinary and Secondary Meridians is felt to be ruled by a different "Patron" of treatment that is outside the scope of Five Element acupuncture. It is believed that Five Element treatment and the other special methods included in LA can achieve the same results, without needing to resort to these other Patrons which are part of a different tradition.

4) CAUSES OF DISEASE: Disease can occur only when one or more of the Officials is malfunctioning. This can occur as a result of either external or internal factors. The external factors are essentially the perverse climatic conditions while the internal factors are the extremes of emotional trauma referred to earlier. Worsley teaches that within his own lifetime he has seen the predominant etiological mechanism change from the external factors when he was younger to the internal ones operative today when most people have adequate food, clothing and shelter, yet still get just as sick as did their grandparents. There is also a miscellaneous category of factors which relates to trauma, constitutional weaknesses, and above all, unhealthy lifestyles. These relate to diet, exercise, sexuality and other more spiritual aspects of life that will perforce lead to illness if they are not conducted according to the Laws of Nature by which we are all maintained.

5) DISEASE PROCESSES: Although all disease ultimately reflects malfunctioning Officials, the mechanisms preventing their normal functioning can vary. The simplest diseases occur when an Official becomes habitually overactive or underactive. Since all activity is dependent on the same Qi, usually when one Official is overactive (appropriating too much Qi) it will be at the expense of some other Official which, deprived of its normal share of Qi, will become underactive. This

"normal" process of illness is the kind ideally suited to Five Element treatment, however there are other types of disease process which obstruct Five Element acupuncture from working properly, and in LA must be treated first. The simplest of these cases is the existence of a blockage in the flow of Qi along the Meridians. This blockage can be either between the left and right halves of a Meridian (called an Akabane imbalance), between one Meridian and the following Meridian along the "Wei circuit" (called an Entry–Exit block), or along the midline Extrameridians (called a GV–CV block). More serious kinds of disease mechanism that demand priority in treatment include Possession, Aggressive Energy (AE) and Husband/Wife imbalance (H/W). Possession describes a situation where the patient is no longer in control of his own Qi. It can be thought of either as a situation of being controlled by some outside force or "devil" or alternatively as one of being controlled by an internal compulsion or obsession—the important point is that an abnormal energetic pattern has taken over some level of the patient's functioning—Body, Mind or Spirit. Serious cases of Possession can be found among patients classified as insane, but less severe examples can be found in people who can exist in society, without ever knowing what it is like to feel all right in themselves. Aggressive Energy, or AE is a polluted form of Qi that is poisoning one or more of the Officials. Again it can come from an external or an internal source, but as long as it is present, Five Element treatment is contraindicated, as it may spread this polluted energy. AE is both diagnosed and treated via the AEP's (Back Shu Points). The final disease mechanism that can occur, a Husband/Wife imbalance, is felt to be the most dangerous. An H/W represents a situation where the patient's own self-healing mechanisms are shutting down, reflecting a turning away from Natural Law. This usually occurs in response to a truly catastrophic situation in someone's life, and it reflects a breakdown of the most fundamental Law of Yin/Yang balance. The H/W is diagnosed from the pulses, (those on the right wrist being excesive with respect to those on the left wrist) and treated by a protocol to re-establish Yin/Yang balance. A final aspect of disease process which is relatively unique to LA is the teaching that diseases evolve in a specific direction and sequence, and that in healing, the symptoms will temporarily reoccur in the reverse order. This is known as the "Law of Cure."

6) CLINICAL EXAMINATION: Traditionally, examination entails four aspects: seeing, hearing (which in Chinese includes smelling), questioning and feeling. These are not unique to LA, but two aspects are: Firstly, all information to be gathered in the examination is felt to reflect the Elements or Officials whose state of health and balance is itself being examined, and secondly, examination findings are only considered to be reliable if the patient allows his true situation to be

exposed. This can only occur if there is good rapport with the patient which builds on trust, thus developing rapport is the most consistently practiced examination skill in Leamington—not pulse diagnosis nor any of the other technical skills. The Five Element information of greatest value is the subtle color which appears on the temples and other areas of the face, the patient's vocal quality and odor, and finally the emotion which predominates inappropriately when the patient is under stress. These four findings are called Color, Sound, Odor and Emotion, and are felt to be the only reliable basis for evaluating the cause of imbalance amongst the Five Elements. Although easily described in a single sentence, the skill involved in perceiving them accurately can take a lifetime to master, as they are both subtle reflections of energetic phenomena and also easily disguised by the social masks we all adopt in order to be seen in the "most favorable light." Other details of the LA examination that are relatively unique include the method and interpretation of the radial artery twelve position pulse diagnosis, which is carried out while holding the patient's hand to facilitate rapport, while the palpating hand uses only the very tips of the fingers held perpendicular to the artery. The volumes of the pulses at each of the positions (recorded as gradations of plus and minus) is learned first while the pulse qualities are considered to be material for post-graduate study. The changes in the pulse are of paramount importance in the conduct of the acupuncture treatment and so they will always be felt before and after each treatment and perhaps several times in between. Other specific areas for examination include the abdomen, musculoskeletal structure and heat sensitivity at the ends of the Meridians (Akabane test), but really every aspect of each patient's being—from the way they walk to the color of their socks—is felt to express something about their inner selves, and is used diagnostically. Worsley at one time described teaching "diagnosis at a glance" by having his students watch passengers getting off railway trains and from this simple observation try to assess their Elemental state. A final detail about the LA asking or history taking process is that the important part is to write down the exact words of the patient, for it is often the manner of expression and not the content per se which is of most significance.

7) TRADITIONAL DIAGNOSIS: There is one primary aim in making an LA diagnosis and that is to correctly identify the Causative Factor or CF of the patient's energetic imbalance. The CF is one of the Five Elements which has been damaged in its functioning to such a degree that it produces a constant state of imbalance which does not change over time. The CF is identified by Color, Sound, Odor and Emotion, and is the primary focus of acupuncture treatment, which is why LA is colloquially referred to as Five Element acupuncture. Having identified the CF, it is also important to identify the level of disease—is it primarily

due to malfunction of the Body, the Mind or the Spirit? Knowing the level can provide the key to choosing the most effective points for treatment. In a similar way, knowing the imbalanced Element within the Element of the CF can also be useful, but is again considered to be a post-graduate issue. After identifying the CF, blocks and other special conditions such as Possession, AE and H/W must be identified. The remaining issue with regard to both diagnosis and treatment in LA is that it is not symptom oriented. This means that the nature of the symptom does not inform the LA practitioner about the energetic cause which created it, and therefore provides no rational guide to diagnosis or treatment. LA dogma states quite literally that any symptom can be caused by any one of the Five Elements and thus cannot help us understand the energetic mechanism at fault. This teaching is diametrically opposed to that of TCM which is specifically oriented towards interpreting and treating the symptoms.

8) TREATMENT: I like to call the method of transferring Qi from Meridians in Excess to those in Deficiency through the Five Element cycles and Command Points, the "Central Dogma" of LA. It is practically the first treatment principle taught in LA, but it is rarely encountered in other styles of acupuncture. LA treatment also makes use of other Command Points such as the Source and Horary Points which are felt to be the safest to use, and special Points used for their "Spirits" such as the "Windows of the Sky." In general, the treatment is focussed on improving the functional state of the Officials of the CF and this is usually done by transferring Qi into them or otherwise Tonifying them if they are Deficient, which is usually the case. In a minority of patients the treatment required will be Sedation or Dispersion, but this is governed by the findings on pulse diagnosis. Tonification is accomplished by a rapid needle technique that only takes a moment, while Sedation requires leaving the needles in place for from several minutes to an hour at times. Each treatment is different depending on the energetic diagnosis at the time, and usually Tonification is the method of choice to begin with and is preferentially applied on the patient's left side, while Sedation is preferentially applied on the patient's right side. Relatively few Points are used in each treatment which along with the forementioned aspects of technique differentiate LA from other styles of acupuncture. Contrarywise, some aspects of LA treatment are common in other styles: situations when treatment is forbidden (drunkenness, exhaustion, etc,), the use of First-Aid or Emergency Points, and other special Points such as the Seas and Oceans. There are two final comments I have about LA treatment. The first is that there is a special emphasis on treating the Heart Protector and Three Heater Officials which are felt to be almost universally imbalanced, even in patients who do not have the Fire Element as their CF. Finally, treatment in LA is not

caried out with the needles alone, nor only with the accompanying techniques such as moxibustion, important as it is. Once again, the rapport established with the patient enables the practitioner to become a part of the treatment itself, and this aspect of therapy is emphasized. The practitioner is felt to be a "vehicle" through which the healing power of Nature can be re-introduced, and a good practitioner uses not only physical tools but also compassion and guidance to help his patients back on the road to health.

Having now reviewed the essential teachings of LA, let me return to the quest for its roots. Since I've already established that it is a syncretic approach, the first task in trying to reconstruct its development would obviously be to identify Worsley's sources of information— his own teachers and other influences.

Partly with the goal of verifying the historical validity of the material I studied under him, and partly just to satisfy my own curiosity, I have, from the time I began studying with Worsley in 1973, attempted to find out these sources for his teachings. Although the following narrative is written somewhat in the form of a detective story of how I pried into my "master's" somewhat shadowy past, it is at the same time a continuation of the previous chapter, and although it focuses on one branch of Oriental medicine, LA, which is, I think possibly, the least well-known and the most poorly documented branch, my goal is a larger one: to describe the outlines at least of the whole living tree, to which it is organically attached.

On several occasions, I was able to talk briefly with Worsley about his own training, and I can summarize the salient features as follows: He had two main teachers, Masters Ono from Japan and Hsu[245] from China, both of whom he met and studied with at International Acupuncture Conferences, mainly in Germany, intermittently over a period of time. Both of them purportedly practiced essentially the same style of acupuncture as that which Worsley teaches, and he transmits to his students what his mentors told him—that this style is the classical method of acupuncture handed down by oral tradition from antiquity. I have in my research, discovered three other interviews in which Worsley has spoken about his training which essentially corroborate the history I obtained, with the additional mention of an unnamed German doctor who was credited with being a formative influence in one of the interviews.[246] This is clearly, however, the barest of skeletons as far as professional biographies go, and accounts for my description of his past as "shadowy." The fact that no one else I interviewed for the first fifteen years of my research had ever heard of Ono or Hsu only added to the mystery, and explains the "detective story" format of this presentation. Of course, it is well-known that Professor Worsley visited the Orient, and photographs have been published showing him spending time with many prominent practitioners such as C.Y. Chen (Fig.93), and Lok Yee-Kung (Fig.94) in Hong Kong, and Wu Wei-p'ing (Figs.95A and B—we see him in figure 95 being confounded with his travelling companion, Malcolm Stemp) in Taiwan, but Professor Worsley has not publicly described these people as his "teachers" and so the presumption has been that he met them after having already been trained. Be that as it may, Worsley and Stemp did formally request training and patronage from Wu Wei-p'ing in 1966 as can be seen in Figures 96 through 102.[247] I have also mentioned in Chapter Four Worsley's visit to James Tin Yau So (Fig.103), and could add other Chinese teachers, such as Leung Kok-yuen whom Worsley visited, but never described as his teacher. Which brings me back to the mystery of Ono, Hsu, and the German doctor, none of whom appear in photographs with Worsley, nor were even identifiable by any of his colleagues, but all of whom can be expected to re-enter the story as it unfolds.

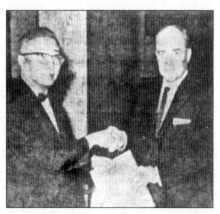

Figure 93: WORSLEY AND CHEN CHAN-YUEN IN HONG KONG, 1966. Professor Chen's writings on Chinese medical history are cited in the bibliography.

For the moment, let me reiterate that all of my early attempts to make sense of Worsley's story, and to follow-up on it, came to naught. I interviewed Wu Wei-p'ing in Taiwan and many of the pioneers of acupuncture in England, including the late Harry Cadman (Fig.104), the first President of the Traditional Acupuncture Society (TAS) who had been practicing acupuncture in England since the 1930's, and the late Denis Lawson-Wood (Fig.105), author of the

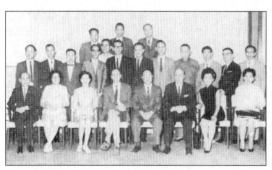

Figure 94: THE KOWLOON COLLEGE OF ACUPUNCTURE IN HONG KONG, 1966. The head of the College, Lok Yee-Kung (see Figure 89), is flanked by Worsley on the right and Malcolm Stemp on the left.

first coherent book about acupuncture in English, and an early colleague of Worsley's, without hearing a hint of the sources cited. I also essentially struck out in this regard, in a brief correspondence before he died in 1987, with Jacques Lavier (Fig.106), the French acupuncturist who translated and popularized Wu Wei-p'ing's work, and introduced the study of the Five Elements and energy transfers via the Creative and Control cycles into England in his 1963 seminars, which were attended by Worsley and many of the other pioneers of British acupuncture, including Royston Low (Fig.107) of the British Acupuncture Association (BAA) and Dick Van Buren (Fig.108) of the International College of Oriental Medicine (ICOM).

Actually, I had gotten to the point where I felt I had reached a dead-end, and had stopped actively pursuing these loose ends, when I came upon a most interesting piece of writing which got me started once again. The following are some quotations of passages from a French text that I happened upon in the library of the University of California, San Francisco:[248]

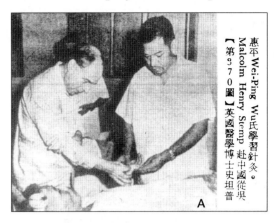

A

惠平 Wei-Ping Wu 氏學習針灸。
Malcolm Henry Stemp 赴中國從吳
【第 370 圖】英國醫學博士史坦普

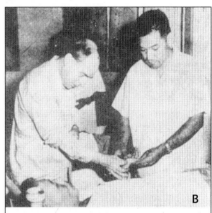

B

【第 158 圖】英國醫學博士華禮士 Dr. J.R Worlsey 赴中國從吳惠平 Wei-Ping Wu 氏學習針灸。

Figure 95: WORSLEY IN CLINIC WITH WU WEI P'ING

in Taipei, 1966. (A) Chen's caption misidentifies Worsley as Stemp. (B) Hsu's republication corrected this error.

("Man is nourished by) . . . three sorts of food: solids and liquids, air, sensations and their associated thoughts."[249]

"Observation, one of the 4 methods of diagnosis, allows the possibility of completely knowing the patient from a single glance! His present state as well as his past and future."[250]

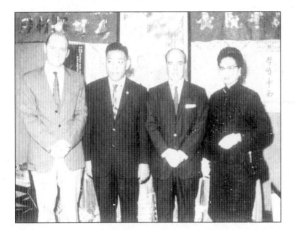

Figure 96:

From left to right (for the following series, all from Worsley's 1966 visit to Taiwan)

MALCOLM STEMP, WU WEI-P'ING, WORSLEY, MRS. WU.

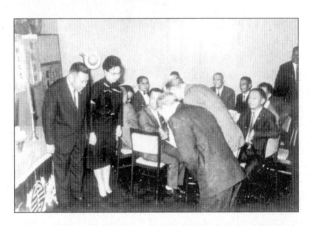

Figure 97: WORSLEY AND STEMP bow to Professor and Mrs. Wu.

Figure 98:

WORSLEY AND STEMP bow to a portrait of Wu's parents, part of the ritual of discipleship. Eric Tao (the translator) smiles in the background as Wu acknowledges the bow.

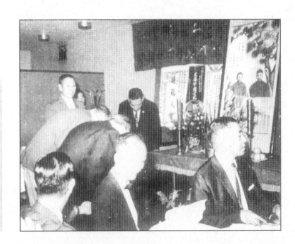

Figure 99:

WU DEMONSTRATES
FACIAL NEEDLING

technique as Worsley observes. (The Point being stimulated appears to be Bladder-1, which Worsley later personally needled on all of his students as part of their training. Moxa on the handle of a needle is seen on the patient's forearm.)

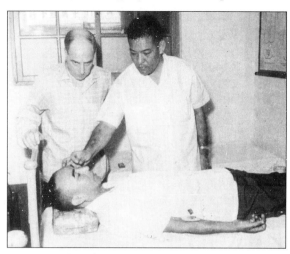

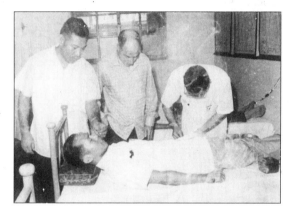

Figure 100:
Wu's assistant lights the moxa needles at Small Intestine-3 as Wu needles another facial Point and Worsley observes.

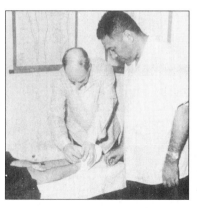

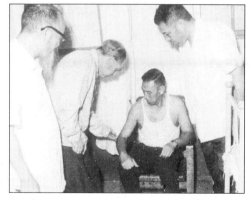

Figure 101:
Worsley inserts moxa needles along the Stomach Meridian under Wu's guidance.

Figure 102:
Worsley applies moxa to the needles along the Large Intestine Meridian as Wu and his assistant Wang observe.

("By training your powers of observation and intuition). . . you will discover all sorts of abnormalities in people who believe themselves to be physically and morally healthy. You can determine the stage or depth of the illness, evaluate the degree of physical, physiological, mental or spiritual disease. This latter category of illness is the hardest to cure, but unfortunately it's very widespread. Spiritual blindness is a much worse affliction than mere physical blindness."[251]

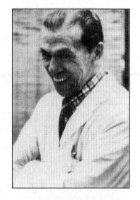

"The greater circulation (as opposed to the GV/CV small circulation) of defensive energy (Wei Qi) is the superficial one of the 12 meridians, from Lung . . . to Liver."[252]

"One feels the superficial pulse by lightly touching the tip of the finger to the pulse position and then gently increasing the pressure. For the deep pulse, one starts by completely compressing the artery, then slightly relaxing the pressure."[253]

Figure 103: Dr. James Tin Yau So, founder of the New England School of Acupuncture, was trained in the lineage of Cheng Dan-an —see Footnote 231.

"Certain of the pulses can be more or less big or more or less small. Some may even be missing. You should note these as follows: "O" is an equilibrated pulse, "-" is a small, shrunken pulse, "+" is a big, full, overflowing pulse. "+ and -" indicate the size of the pulse and not its force. A "+" pulse can be weak or strong, hard or soft—the same for a "-" pulse. "-" pulses indicate lack of energy, (Yin state), therefore one tonifies. "+" pulses indicate excess of of energy, (Yang state), therefore one disperses.[254]

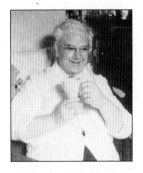

Figure 104:

Harry Cadman, one of the earliest practitioners to use acupuncture in the U.K., was on the faculty of the College of Chinese Acupuncture in Oxford while the author was in attendance. He learned acupuncture in 1932 from a colonial doctor (Pakes) who had worked in the Far East.

"If there is deficiency in an organic system (Official) that's a Yin state. One must tonify or call to make the energy come there."[255]

"Theoretically, if your diagnosis has been done correctly, 1 or 2 needles are sufficient for each treatment. One should always use the least number of needles possible. Hua Tuo was famous 19 centuries ago for only using one needle per treatment, which is the ideal. The *"Zhen Jiu I Xue"* of 1798 said, "a single needle can cure hundreds of maladies. Use at most 4 needles. Those who fill the body with needles are detestable."[256]

"If you can't remember these 12 points, which are so pre-cious, you only need to learn the following 6 points which you tonify or disperse according to the disequilibrium. (H8, Liv. 1, K10, L8, Sp3, Cx 8)"(257)

"Don't treat pregnant women. . . Don't treat during periods of bad weather—tempest, storms, very hot weather, or at full moon."(258)

"To tonify, turn the needle to restore skin tone and quickly remove the needle and close the hole. This only takes a few seconds. To tonify it is best to use points on the left side of the body."(259)

"To disperse, turn the needle to get it in to the desired depth, and leave it there till the skin relaxes. Then withdraw it gen-tly and slowly, and leave the hole open. This may take 10 to 30 minutes. It is best to disperse points on the right side of the body."(260)

"After (needling) one must verify that the corresponding pulses have returned to normal."(261)

"Tonification reinforces the energy of a single organic func-tion (Official) while dispersion, by the diffusion of energy it provokes, produces a tonification of the whole organism. . . In treatment, tonification should always come first, and one should never tonify and disperse at the same time in the first several sessions. Dispersion should be reserved for the end of the treatment sequence. For each session, one or two points should be used, and treat from once to three times a week according to the gravity of the illness."(262)

One should never try to simply eliminate (the patient's) suf-fering, pain or other symptoms. . . Symptomatic treatment is actually complicity in the original violation of natural law which was responsible for the problem in the first place."(263)

I've reproduced these passages at length especially for the bene-fit of those trained at Leamington who will most likely hear in them the echoes of Professor Worsley himself. When I first read these quotes to a group of Leamington graduates, the majority opinion was that he must have been the author. In fact, the original manuscript from which these quotations were derived was written by Sakurazawa Nyoitchi in the late 1950's and the actual source text quoted was a contorted ver-sion of this manuscript which was published posthumously in 1969.(264) Sakurazawa was more popularly known by his Westernized name, George Ohsawa (1893–1966), and he was the originator of Macrobiotics, a shoot off the trunk of Oriental medicine using mainly dietary therapy guided by a highly idiosyncratic version of Yin-Yang theory (Fig.109). The book I've quoted from translates into English as *"Acupuncture and the Medicine of the Far East."*

The story of macrobiotics itself provides an interesting diversion into the cross connections between various Eastern and Western approaches to natural healing which I would like to mention briefly, as this topic will be a recurrent one.[265] Ohsawa had been interested in Oriental medicine ever since as a young man he cured himself of tuberculosis—an illness which had already killed others in his family—by experimenting with dietary practices recommended by a Japanese physician, Ishizuka Sagen (1850–1910) (Fig.110). Ishizuka had developed his own dietary theories after years of self-experimentation in grappling with chronic kidney disease. Though he was influenced by the classics of Oriental medicine, he believed equally strongly in Western science, and his system boiled down to an attempt to explain all illness as resulting from a dietarily derived deviation in the normal potassium/sodium balance in the body. He called his approach "shoku-yo," which means "nutritional" or "food-cure" and he was colloquially known as Dr. Miso Soup and Dr. Daikon. In spite of these epithets, Ishizuka was immensely popular, and had to limit his consultations to only one hundred per day! Ohsawa popularized and developed Ishizuka's ideas, and re-injected an Oriental as opposed to Western medical credo by choosing Yin/Yang rather than potassium/sodium balance as the foundation, but as I mentioned, his interpretation of Yin/Yang was idiosyncratic and differs, for example, from the use of Yin and Yang in TCM. Ohsawa was continually shuttling back and forth between Eastern and Western modes of thought and terminology. In 1947, at the same time that he Westernized his own name, George Ohsawa chose the word "macrobiotics" to describe his version of Oriental medicine, but he borrowed the term from a Western medical treatise, *Macrobiotics or the Art of Prolonging Human Life* by the German Christoph Wilhelm Hufeland (1762–1836) (Fig.111). Macrobiotics was in turn coined by Hufeland from the Greek roots for "great-all-embracing" and "life." Hufeland, as a physician, was searching for a sounder basis for medical practice, and believed it was to be found in the cultivation of the "life-force" (die Lebenskraft). This life-force is clearly parallel to the Chinese concept of Qi as it was traditionally envisioned, complete with both material and spiritual aspects. It was a concept which Hufeland shared with his friend and colleague, Dr. Samuel Hahnemann (1775–1843), the founder of homeopathy (Fig.112). As an aside, I might note that the disciple of Hahnemann who brought homeopathy to America, Constantine Hering[266] (Fig.113) (1800–1880) (who was also the first physician to use nitro-glycerine for angina), was the originator of the "Law of Cure" taught as part of LA, but once again we must wait to dis-

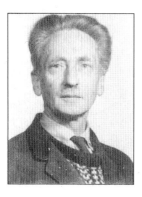

Figure 105: Denis Lawson-Wood, co-author with his wife Joyce of a dozen books about acupuncture including the seminal *Chinese System of Healing* in 1959, and President of the British Acupuncture Association from 1969 to 1970.

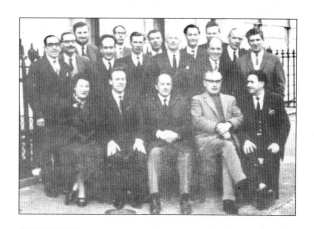

Figure 106: Jacques Lavier, surrounded by the graduates of his historic 1963 London seminar. From left to right they are, rear row: Bill Wright, Keith Lamont, Paul Gill, Shyam Singha, Dick Van Buren and Bob Butterworth; middle row: Eli Cohen, Royston Low, George Pandellis, Gerald Lancaster, Val Winsor, Jack Worsley and John Sugarman; front row: Jean Gill, Ken Underhill, Jacques Lavier, Bob Challis and one unidentified graduate.

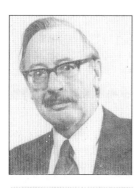

Figure 107: Royston Low, former President of the British Acupuncture Association and Dean of the British College of Acupuncture.

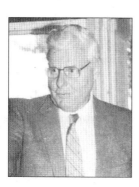

Figure 108: J.D. (Dick) van Buren, Founder and former Principal of the International College of Oriental Medicine and Director of the International Register of Oriental Medicine.

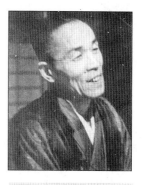

Figure 109: George Ohsawa (1893–1966), also known as Sakurazawa Nyoitchi or Sakurazawa Yukikazu, was the originator of Macrobiotics. He also wrote numerous books and articles which introduced many aspects of Japanese culture to Europe for the first time.

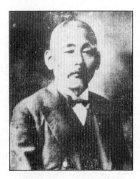

Figure 110: ISHIZUKA SAGEN (1850– 1910), the Japanese physician whose nutritional approach to disease, called "Shoku-yo," was the forerunner of Macrobiotics.

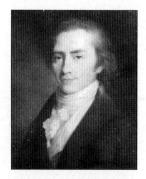

Figure 111: CHRISTOPH WILHELM HUFELAND (1762–1836) the German physician of the vitalist school who coined the term Macrobiotics.

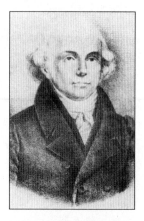

Figure 112: SAMUEL HAHNEMANN (1775–1843), the German physician who founded homeopathy in response to what he perceived as the inadequacies of conventional medicine, an approach which he called allopathy.

cover how this medical dogma found its way from a German physician practicing in the United States to an English practitioner of an Asian style of medicine. Returning to Hufeland, his many works were translated into Japanese in the 1800's and "his name became familiar to many who had never learned a foreign language. His reputation was widespread and he was regarded as the most important authority on the treatment of cholera, which in 1858 spread for the first time over the entire Japanese kingdom,"[267] thus it is not strange that Ohsawa would have been familiar with Hufeland's work. Hufeland was also the personal physician of the romantic poet Goethe, who, in his most famous work *Faust* sounded the rallying cry of the vitalists against those holding to the materialist philosophy typical of Western medicine even in the eighteenth century:

> "He who would study organic existence,
> First drives out the soul with rigid persistence
> Then the parts in his hand he may hold and class
> But the spiritual link is lost alas."[268]

Thus, by tapping into the vitalistic traditions of both the East and the West, George Ohsawa taught an approach to medicine that had as many adherents in one of these worlds as in the other, and it is not so surprising that many of his ideas parallel those of Worsley. I will return to Ohsawa in another context at the end of this story, but for now I'd like to describe my search for a substantive basis for the common ideas of these two charismatic teachers, a task which was nowhere near as easy as I had hoped it might be.

I made extensive studies to see if Worsley had ever had any contact with Ohsawa, who died in 1966, which would explain the similarity of their teachings, but met with negative results from every source including Ohsawa's American biographer, Ron Kotzsch, his most serious archivist, Dr. Marc Van Cauwenbergh, and many of the leaders of the macrobiotic movement in the U.S. and abroad (including Clim Yoshimi, Jacques de Langre, Shizuko Yamamoto, William Dufty, Bill Tara and Michio Kushi). Two macrobiotic students from Worsley's second American class (1973) (Michael Rosoff and Robert Gerzon) both reported that Professor Worsley was at that time actively hostile to the idea of macrobiotics, and I can confirm that from my own Licentate class, where Worsley described his insistence that a prospective macro-

biotic patient eat a hamburger before he would agree to treat him. Worsley did, however, lecture in the early 70's in Boston, under Michio Kushi's sponsorship (see Fig.114 for a momento of that visit) and Kushi was responsible for encouraging his students to study with Worsley. Kushi (Fig.115) himself, later (1973) wrote about acupuncture and lectured in London under the auspices of the BAA and Sidney Rose-Neil, but his teachings bear no resemblance to the excerpts I quoted from Ohsawa, nor did the teachings of the only other Japanese macrobiotic acupuncturist of prominence living in the West, Noborou Muramoto (Fig.116) who wrote the popular text *Healing Ourselves*. Under Kushi's guidance, an English translation of Ohsawa's acupuncture teachings was produced,[269] but it is more of a ghost-written work than a translation, and bears

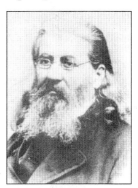

Figure 113: CONSTANTINE HERING (1800–1880), the German-American disciple of Hahnemann who originated the "Law of Cure."

no resemblance to Worsley's teachings, so Kushi can be eliminated as an explanation of the Worsley/Ohsawa link. The best connection between these two which I have managed to discover consists of several rather tenuous links. The first is via Denis Lawson-Wood (1906–1990) who studied with Ohsawa in England between 1960 and 1962, and who was a colleague of Worsley from 1962 on, however very little of Lawson-Wood's published material, which is voluminous, mentions either the focus on the Spirit or the technical material quoted from *Acupuncture and the Medicine of the Far East* which is so reminiscent of LA. This latter publication wasn't even done until 1969 (although it dealt with events in 1958) by which time Lawson-Wood had stopped studying with Ohsawa and also stopped close contact with Worsley (who had started his own school in 1966). The second, more promising but still indirect link turns out to be one of the candidates for the role of the mysterious German doctor who was actually present at the class in 1958 on which Ohsawa's book was based.[270] His identity was only revealed at the tail-end of my attempts to follow the two leads given in Ohsawa's book, and so he shall remain anonymous a while longer. The first lead was Ohsawa's mention of a collaboration with Soulié de Morant (Fig.117) in 1934, co-translating a Japanese work by T. Nakayama, *"Acupuncture and Chinese Medicine Verified in Japan."* In this endeavor, Ohsawa did the bulk of the translation, and Soulié de Morant handled the technical terms, so it would appear that Ohsawa's knowledge of acupuncture was still elementary in 1934. In the late 1950's text he mentions that the clinical material was contributed by Mme. Hashimoto (Fig.118), a Japanese practitioner who co-presented a series of classes with Ohsawa in Europe in 1958, on which experience his treatise was based (Fig.119 and 120).

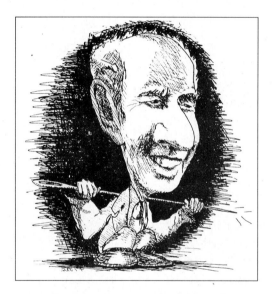

Figure 114: INTERVIEW WITH JACK WORSLEY in "The East West Journal," June 30, 1972, conducted in Boston, where he was teaching a seminar.

So now we have two leads to follow: Soulié de Morant and Hashimoto. Each will take us down a separate but fruitful path. Let's start with Soulié de Morant, as he was chronologically prior.

I think we can say that contemporary traditional acupuncture in the West, whatever that is, started with George Soulié de Morant, (1878 –1955) in 1927 in France. Prior to that date, there had been scattered accounts and even some books about acupuncture in Western languages, but no attempt to formulate a systematic energetic understanding of acupuncture based on Points, Meridians, the circulation of Qi and its management and reflection in pulse diagnosis had ever been attempted.

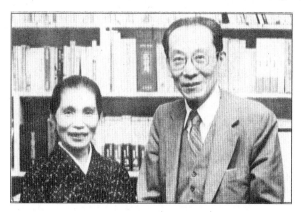

Figure 115: MICHIO KUSHI AND HIS WIFE AVELINE Kushi came to the United States in 1949 as Ohsawa's emissary under the sponsorhip of Norman Cousins. He has been the most vocal proponent of Macrobiotics since Ohsawa's death.

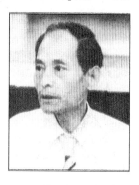

Figure 116: NOBORU MURAMOTO, author of the popular Macrobiotics text *Healing Ourselves*. He taught acupuncture to students in California in the mid-1970's.

Soulié de Morant[(271)] grew up in an unusual family that encouraged him to learn Chinese from the tender age of eight. He was originally schooled by the Jesuits, and like many of the people I will mention in this chapter, intended to study medicine, but had to give up that ambition when his father died. At 21, based on his linguistic skills, he got a secretarial job in China, and happened to be in Peking during a cholera epidemic, which is an acute illness with a high mortality (usually 30 to 50%). Soulié de Morant made the acquaintance of a Dr. Yang, who was extraordinarily successful in treating cholera victims with acupuncture (using more or less a formula treatment: S25, S36, LI10 and Points around CV8) and Soulié de Morant's curiosity was piqued, to the point that he began studying with Dr. Yang, who even let him do some of these treatments under his guidance.

As an aside, it is of interest that the treatment of cholera and other epidemics which I have already mentioned in connection with Hufeland's reputation in Japan, was also a field in which homeopathy made notable advances, a parallel history to which I would like to return

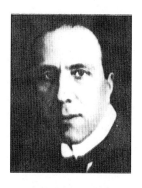

Figure 117: GEORGE SOULIÉ DE MORANT (1878–1955), the "Grandfather" of traditional acupuncture in the West, he was a prolific author, publishing over twenty books and articles about acupuncture. The publication of his magnum opus, *Chinese Acupuncture*, led to his nomination for the Nobel Prize in physiology in 1950, but the prize was ultimately won by scientists from Switzerland and America.

later. Homeopathic camphor was actually considered to be a specific treatment for cholera by Hahnemann, who discovered this connection.

Soulié de Morant was subsequently appointed to the French Consular Corps and sent to various cities in China, in each of which he sought out acupuncture teachers—a Dr. Zhang in Shanghai and several unnamed doctors in Yunnan being prominent. I should point out that Yunnan province is contiguous with Indochina, including Vietnam, and it is likely that the initial Vietnamese influence on French acupuncture is probably a consequence of Soulié de Morant's studies in Yunnan. Soulié de Morant was unusual in that he adopted local custom as his own, and it was said that when he dressed up, his speech and manner were indistinguishable from a native Chinese, and so he earned the respect and trust of his teachers, who supplied him with the most precious texts and instruction. He became so proficient a practitioner, that in 1908 the Viceroy of Yunnan certified him as a "Master Physician-Acupuncturist"—quite an extraordinary honor (Fig.121).

One other Oriental influence on Soulié de Morant came from Japan, where he spent a month in 1906 because of his own poor state of health, and is reflected in Soulié de Morant's later citation of Japanese works in his publications. Thus, we can see that from its very inception, the European acupuncture which Soulié de Morant inaugurated, reflected aspects of Chinese, Japanese and Vietnamese tradition. In fact, Soulié de Morant also cited several classical Korean texts, so that tradition was represented, too. Soulié de Morant was an extraordinary individual, whose work encompassed many fields: art, literature, music, theater, linguistics and history, but there is no room here to discuss his accomplishments in those areas. However, let me just mention one curious historical incident that may have had a tremendous impact on world history: during his tenure as Vice-Consul in Yunnan in 1908, Soulié de Morant had occasion to help Sun Yat-Sen (Fig.122) by signing a visa for him which allowed this famous revolutionary father of modern China to escape from the imperial police who were trying to catch him.

Soulié de Morant returned to France in 1918, but it was not until 1927 that his Western career in acupuncture really began. At that time, he brought his daughter for medical treatment to a naturopath who specialized in hydrotherapy—Dr. Paul Ferreyroles. Ferreyroles was a member of a study group of physicians investigating alternative, or what is today called "complementary" medicine (including Drs. Marcel and Thérèse Martiny and later Flandin, Bonnet-Lemaire and Khoubesserian) and they prevailed upon Soulié de Morant to abandon all his other interests, and translate the classical Chinese medical texts into French and train them in acupuncture treatment. This he did, while developing a clinical-experimental practice, first under medical supervision in sev-

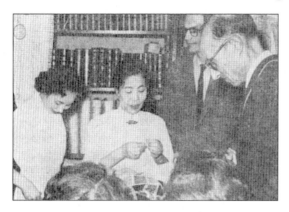

Figure 118:
HASHIMOTO MASAE
(1899–1981) (center)
teaching acupuncture in
France in 1958.

Figure 119: OHSAWA
AND HASHIMOTO
collaboratively teaching
the use of Five Element
theory in acupuncture,
March 26, 1958.

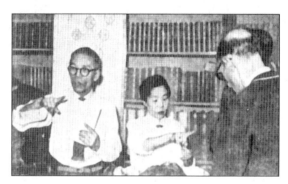

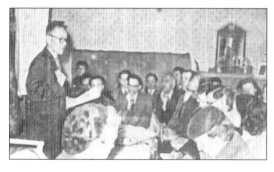

Figure 120: OHSAWA
lecturing on acupunc-
ture, with Honma's
Meridian chart in the
background, 1958.

Figure 121:
SOULIÉ DE MORANT
as a member of the
French Consular Corps in
Shanghai (he's the tallest
of the French).

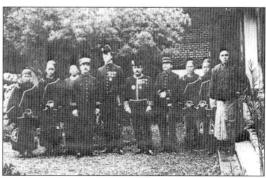

eral hospitals, and later in private practice where he treated among others, the famous literary figure, Antonin Artaud.[272] He also experimented on himself, needling different points to see their effects, and kept careful records which he used in his subsequent publications.

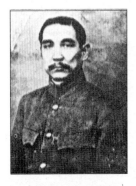

Figure 122:

SUN YAT-SEN

(1866–1925), a physician whose revolutionary activity helped lead to the foundation of the Republic of China and the downfall of the Qing dynasty.

His first writing about acupuncture was an article in the French Homeopathic Journal in 1929, in collaboration with Ferreyroles, and his first serious book about acupuncture, *Précis de la vrai acuponcture chinoise*, was published in 1934. Altogether he wrote over 20 books and articles on acupuncture, his magnum opus being *L'Acuponcture Chinoise*, the first part of which appeared from 1939-41, but which was only published in its entirety posthumously in 1957, and has just been issued in English translation by Paradigm Press in 1994.

Because Soulié de Morant was essentially the first in the field, he got to choose the terminology, and thus we have him to thank for such technical terms as Meridian, Antique Point, Source Point, Five Element Point, Reunion Point, Command Point, Tonification, Dispersion, Spleen-Pancreas function and Circulation-Sex function. His system of acupuncture therapy is beyond the scope of this presentation, but I would like to mention in the following list, some of his ideas which later appeared as components of LA:

1) The goal of treatment is to have all the 12 pulses equal.[273]

2) You must take the pulse before, during and after every treatment—it is the only basis for a science of energetic treatment.

3) Start by tonifying the deficiency using the tonification point (thus based on Five Elements!) and add the source point if necessary. Only disperse later. "Isn't it best to direct the Excess to a Deficient part?"[274] This presages the idea of using the Five Element cycles to "transfer" Qi.

4) Use horary times to enhance the effect of treatments (though Soulié de Morant recommends tonifying in the subsequent two hour period).

5) If treating the Meridians isn't giving the expected effect on the pulse, then use points on GV and CV.

6) The left hand pulses should be slightly stronger than the right hand pulses. "If the husband is weak and the wife is robust, there will be destruction. If the husband is robust and the wife is weak, there will be security."[275]

7) To treat Evil (Xie) Qi, use the Yu points (AEP's) of each Zang organ (possibly referring to Aggressive Energy). [276]

8) He specifically mentions the following "laws": Mother-Son, Husband-Wife, Midday-Midnight, and treatment by Five Elements using the Command points on each Meridian, with the mandatory inclusion of the coupled Meridian of the same Element. [277] This is exactly how Prof. Worsley organized his chart (Fig.123)

9) In the right hand third pulse position (circulation-sex) he identified the deep pulse as the sexual or genital pulse because its strength clearly varied before and after the menses. The middle level he called the circulation pulse.[278] He identified CV 15 as the Alarm (Mo) Point of sexuality.

10) He claimed that effective needling is often hardly perceptible, citing the Japanese experience.

11) He recognized a commonality of acupuncture and homeopathy—a concordance first pointed out by the German Wiehe in 1903, one of whose parents was a missionary in China, and may have been exposed to acupuncture (Fig.124).

Having compiled this list, I should like to point out that in many significant ways, Soulié de Morant's teachings also differed from LA:

1) Although he employed Five Element principles, his energetic paradigm was Yin/Yang. Thus, he interpreted the Mother-Son law as applying primarily to the superficial sequential circulation of the 12 Meridians as opposed to the deep circulation of the Five Elements. His idea was to balance Yin and Yang by the effect of treating any Meridian on its husband or wife, mother or son, midday-midnight associated and coupled Meridians. Tonifying any Meridian, e.g.,would tonify these other Meridians if they were of the same Yin/Yang polarity, but disperse them if they were of opposite polarity.

2) He was quite interested in Western scientific correlations and explanations for traditional acupuncture, and e.g. cited Arndt's Law that "weak stimulation tonifies, strong stimulation disperses" to understand needle techniques, although

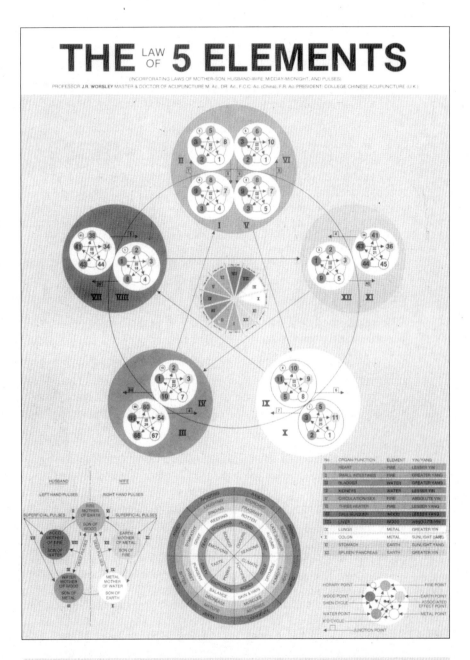

Figure 123: PROFESSOR WORSLEY'S FIVE ELEMENT CHART
THE SMALL PRINT READS, "INCORPORATING LAWS OF MOTHER-SON; HUSBAND-WIFE; MID-DAY-MIDNIGHT; AND PULSES.'

he believed that local and distal points had inverse effects. He advocated using colored versus non-colored metal needles for tonification versus dispersion (probably Vietnamese in origin) based on experiment.[279] He was very interested in the electrical correlates of acupuncture, experimenting with instruments to measure pulses and detect points, and one of his students, Niboyet elaborated extensively on this approach in a 1959 publication.

3) He valued the role of both symptomatic diagnosis and treatment—stressing that the acupuncture points become sensitive in illness and must be searched for using that criterion, and gave treatment formulae for numerous medical conditions and protocols for treating pain itself.

As for Soulié de Morant's sources, aside from his extensive practical training, he used many classical Oriental texts, but his main ones were two Ming dynasty Chinese texts:

1) **ZHEN JIU DA CHENG**—GREAT COMPENDIUM OF ACUPUNCTURE AND MOXIBUSTION (ZJDC) by Yang Ji-zhou (1601). Soulié de Morant was actually confused about the author and dating of this work, attributing it to Yang Ge-xian, although no such individual has been identified by later commentators. Dr. Jean Choain, Soulié de Morant's first biographer, corrected this misattribution in 1978. [280]

2) **YI XUE RU MEN**—THE BASICS OF MEDICAL STUDIES (YXRM) by Li Yan (Li Zhai-jian) (1575). An eight volume text based on a 100 volume text, **GU JIN YI TONG DA QUAN**—ANCIENT AND MODERN MEDICAL WAYS by Xu Chun-fu (1556). Soulié de Morant translated *Basics* as *Le Diagnostic par les Pouls radiaux* which was published with his commentary in 1983, but is not available in English.

Soulié de Morant was also influenced by the Japanese work of Sawada as communicated by Nakayama, whose book he translated into French with Ohsawa. As I mentioned, I will return to Ohsawa and Nakayama from quite a different perspective at the end of this history.

The other source I identified in trying to account for the similarity of Ohsawa's and Worsley's approach to acupuncture was Mme. Hashimoto Masae (1899–1981), who taught with Ohsawa in France in 1958. Her story brings in a whole new lineage, which is much less appreciated in the acupuncture community. How she came to teach in Europe is itself an interesting story.[281] While he was living in Paris in 1957, George Ohsawa decided that acupuncture in France, as derived from the teachings of his former collaborator Soulié de Morant, had gotten off in

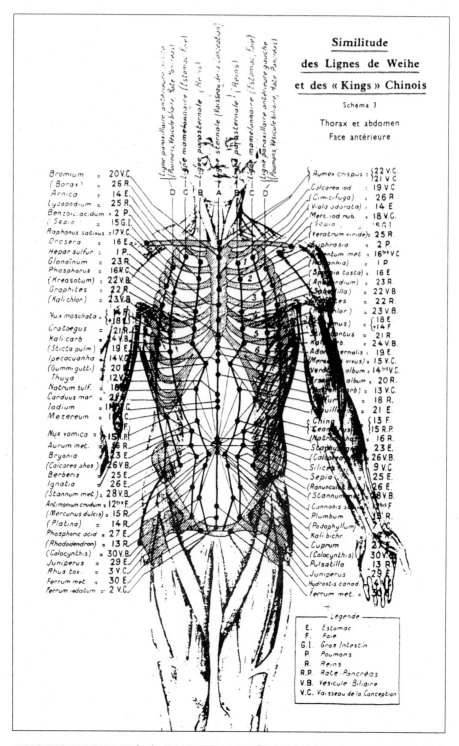

Figure 124: SPONTANEOUSLY TENDER POINTS (POINTS OF WEIHE), their homeopathic indicators, and their correlation with the acupuncture Meridians and Points.

the wrong direction, so he wrote an appeal to the Japanese journal Ido No Nippon for a young but experienced Japanese acupuncturist to come to Paris to help him correct their misguided practice. (It would appear that Ohsawa's main objection to French acupuncture was its lack of focus on the Five Elements, though he himself used Yin/Yang theory exclusively in his dietary therapy!) Mme. Hashimoto was approached by the editors of Ido No Nippon to be the emissary, as she had recently written a series of articles for the Journal on pulse diagnosis (Fig.125), and had a flourishing practice on Nihonbashi in the fashionable Ginza district of Tokyo. The background to this story is that in 1957, a man named Yoneyama Hiroshishu wrote an article claiming that pulse diagnosis was an inaccurate method and so in rebuttal Ido No Nippon sponsored a study of Hashimoto's pulse diagnosis in a clinical setting, and found it to be highly accurate. It is curious though, that her method reversed the pulse positions for men and women, an approach that was at odds with all the other myakushin (pulse diagnosis) practitioners. She additionally emphasized the need to take pulses with the fingertips perpendicularly, and to bend the hand into extension (Fig.126). The nails needed to be clipped extremely short. She was also well-known for her use of moxibustion which she advocated in a book written for the layman (this being an aspect of the Sawada lineage). Her treatments were

Five Element based, but she didn't use "energy transfers" via the Five Element cycles. She simply used the pulses to determine the Excess and Deficient conditions of the 12 Meridians, and then directly treated mainly the Deficient Meridians using Five Element, Alarm and other Command Points with very few needles. She confirmed her diagnoses and monitored her treatments by attending to the following Five Element parameters: color, sound, odor, emotion,

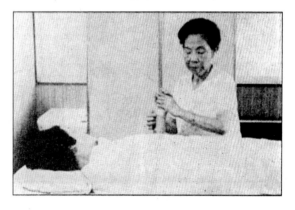

Figure 125: HASHIMOTO'S STYLE OF "PULSE DIAGNOSIS."

An acknowledged master of the art of pulse diagnosis (myakushin), Mme. Hashimoto in fact used a somewhat idiosyncratic technique.

taste preference, sensory function, climatic preference, medical history, and Meridian and abdominal palpation. Her main criterion for an effective treatment was the normalization of the pulse and decrease of abdom-

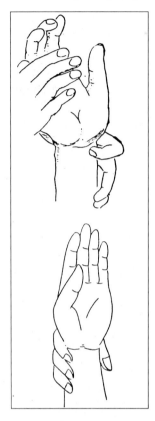

Figure 126:
Correct and incorrect finger placement according to Hashimoto.

inal sensitivity. In keeping track of the lineage and spread of the different traditions, it should be noted that her books and methods were introduced into Taiwan in 1958, which is probably where they were found by Philip Chancellor—the fellow who translated and edited Lavier's version of Wu Wei-p'ing's *Chinese Acupuncture* into English. Hashimoto's original pulse diagnosis articles from Ido No Nippon had been collated by her into a 1961 publication *Japanese Acupuncture*, and it was this work which was translated into English by K. Suzuki and edited by Philip Chancellor for publication in 1968 with the same title. Unfortunately, Chancellor died about two years ago, and Hashimoto herself died in 1981, so the details of her impact on acupuncture in the West are somewhat sketchy. As I indicated, she practiced a very simple Five Element style of treatment, and it is clear that her teachings were the basis for the similarities between Ohsawa and Worsley, though she herself again had no known contact with Professor Worsley! (How Worsley was influenced by Soulié de Morant's teachings also still needs an explanation!) Just as this book was going to press, I did discover a likely lineage for an Ohsawa/Hashimoto to Worsley transmission. A German practitioner from Hamburg, Dr. Elza Munster, who had spent at least two months in clinic with Mme. Hashimoto in Tokyo in 1958 (Fig.127A and B), and who subsequently tutored Nicholas Sofroniou (see Fig.167 to come), one of Worsley's earliest sources of information on acupuncture, seems to have herself had a definite connection to Worsley. Her name appeared sometime after 1967 on a list (see Worsley and Stemp, second edition, in the bibliography) of distinguished Foreign Members of the Acupuncture Guild, a professional organization started by Worsley when he founded his own college. Since Worsley situated his formative acupuncture studies in Germany, there are reasonable grounds to suspect that Dr. Munster played a role in this transmission. She died in 1994 however, so the magnitude of her influence on Worsley is a matter of pure speculation. Curiously, another disciple of Hashimoto, Takenouchi Misao, who had also been close to Ohsawa, visited England with a group of forty macrobiotic students in 1968 (Fig.127C and D). They visited seven European countries as part of the Second World Cultural Olympics, but although Takenouchi gave demonstrations of acupuncture, he did not give any lectures or otherwise engage in teaching, so it is unlikely that any transmission to Worsley would have taken place through him.

Tracing the lineage back one step, Hashimoto had been a nurse who learned the Five Element style of acupuncture from Honma

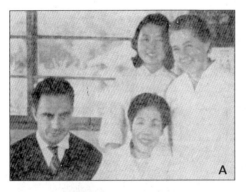

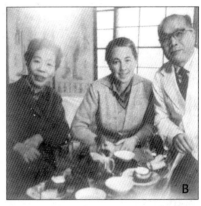

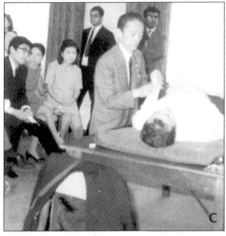

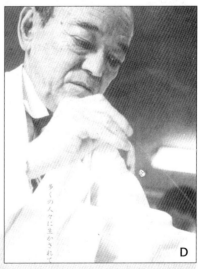

Figure 127:

(A) ELZA MUNSTER (far right) with Mme. Hashimoto (seated). (B) ELZA MUNSTER between Hashimoto and Honma. As a Foreign Member of the Acupuncture Guild affiliated with Worsley's College of Chinese Acupuncture (U.K.), Dr. Munster is in the author's opinion the most likely conduit for the Ohsawa/Hashimoto teachings which Worsley incorporated into LA. (C) TAKENOUCHI MISAO demonstrating acupuncture techniques at the Japanese embassy in London in 1968. (D) TAKENOUCHI MISAO demonstrating his special "piercing" acupuncture technique with long needles. This method is not included in the teachings of LA, so for this and the other reasons indicated in the text, Takenouchi is not a likely source for the Ohsawa/Hashimoto to Worsley transmission, although he was in the right place at the right time.

Shohaku (1904–1962), a very important figure in the revival of classical acupuncture in Japan (Fig.128). His Five Element chart, e.g. (Fig.129) was clearly the basis for the one developed by Worsley. In Figure 128 you can see him lecturing on using the precepts of the *Nan Jing* for pulse diagnosis and treatment. He was a scholar, as well as a practitioner and teacher, and was familiar with classical Korean texts as well as the Chinese and Japanese ones. As a member of the keiraku chiryo (Meridian Therapy) group, his influence, especially on European acupuncturists, was second only to that of the group's founder, his teacher Yanagiya Sorei. Homma died in 1962, just after an important trip to Europe, which I will get to presently. Had he lived a little longer, the course of development of acupuncture in Europe might have been quite different.

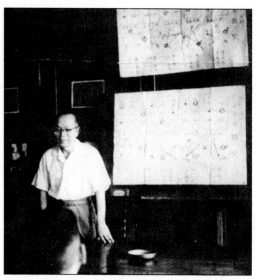

Figure 128: HONMA SHOHAKU (1904–1962), a highly respected teacher of Five Element style acupuncture, is seen here lecturing on the clinical practice of concepts from the *Nan Jing*. Both his Five Element and his Meridian charts are still widely used.

Homma's teacher, as I said, was Yanagiya Sorei[282] (Fig.130) (1906–1959) whose given first name was Seisuke. He changed it to Sorei which is taken from the first words in the titles, *Simple Questions (Su Wen)* and *Vital Axis (Ling Shu)* as a token of his respect for the classics. He was the originator of the revival of Five Element acupuncture in Japan and his students and close colleagues included many famous individuals. You can see the three links in this chain of transmission I've described in Figure 131, a picture taken in 1958, one year before Yanagiya died. To understand Yanagiya's contribution, one needs to know what was happening to acupuncture in Japan in the early 1900's. As reported in the previous chapter, Western medicine had become increasingly popular, and acupuncture began to be co-opted by those with "scientific" training, which culminated in a 1918 government revision of the classification of acupuncture Points

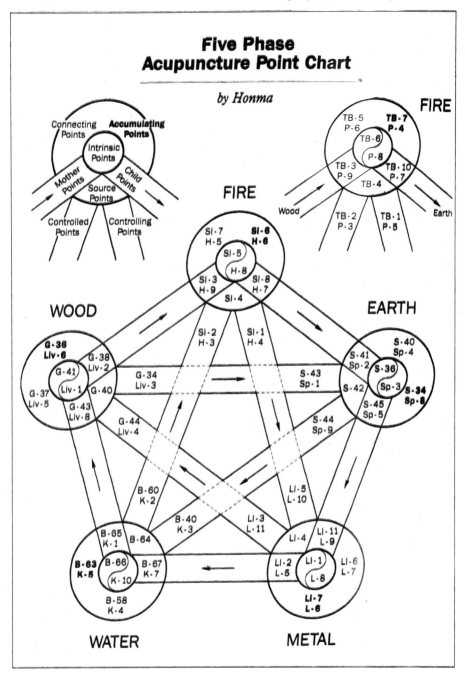

Five Phase Acupuncture Point Chart

by Honma

Figure 129: HONMA'S FIVE ELEMENT CHART.
In form and content, this is clearly the model on which Worsley based his chart (Figure 123).

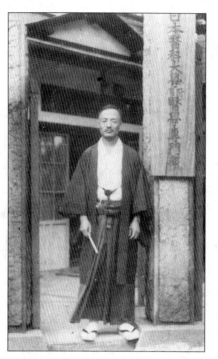

Figure 130: YANAGIYA SOREI (1906–1959), the inspiration behind the revival of Five Element based acupuncture in Japan, which eventuated in keiraku chiryo or Meridian Therapy (MT).

by a topographical grid as opposed to using the traditional Meridian theory. Physicians were required to pass examinations in Western medicine, and there was even an attempt to prohibit traditional medicine outright by the government in 1883. Thus the situation in Japan roughly paralleled what was happening in China, however, the outcome was quite different. Yanagiya, who vigorously opposed the modernizing trend, inspired a generation of Japanese acupuncturists to return to a more classical tradition. As an interesting historical curiosity, Yanagiya not only reinforced the Oriental medical tradition in the practice of acupuncture, but his teachings even impacted the thinking of Dr. Hans Selye, one of the strongest proponents of a more holistic approach to Western medicine as well (Fig.132). In order to comprehend the magnitude of Yanagiya's contribution to Japanese acupuncture per se, and what relationship it might have to LA, a brief review of the history of traditional medicine in Japan is necessary.

As was true for China, the history of medicine in Japan starts in mythological times, and once again has its roots in a shamanistic tradition, which in Japan developed as Shinto, or "the Way of the Spirit." Two legendary figures, Okuninushi-no-mikoto and Sukunahikona-no-mikoto, were said to have discovered the means of curing disease.[283] These included sacrifices, prayers, exorcisms, magical incantations and the like, since diseases were regarded as the work of malign spirits. However, in order for a person to be susceptible to such "possession," he would first have to have transgressed in some way such as unchastity, carelessness, etc. The outcome of all transgressions was "pollution" and the prototypical treatment was the Great Purification ritual (o-harai) which involved the standard shamanistic linking of the three levels: the High Plain of Heaven where the gods (kami) dwell, the world known to man, and the polluted netherworld.[284] Although once the medicine of systematic correspondence was introduced from China, religious healing became less prominent, it never died out, and in particular the majority of the early twentieth century practitioners of acupuncture were steeped in Shinto tradition.[285] There is a popular saying that "Japanese are born into Shinto, get married in Shinto shrines, are buried with Buddhist rituals, and have their lives governed by Confucian social ethics."[286] In fact, new religions have developed in Japan specifically around healing ministries derived from Shinto roots. For example, Tenrikyo, which originated in 1838, teaches that "physical problems originate in the mind and that moral misdeeds (for example,

anger, hatred and avarice) are root causes of personal problems such as illness... (which) is not just something requiring medical treatment, but also spiritual action . . . illness is. . .a sign that one's life has got out of balance and needs reform."[287] There is an obvious similarity between this point of view and the doctrines of LA concerning both the importance of the Spirit and the possibility of possession.

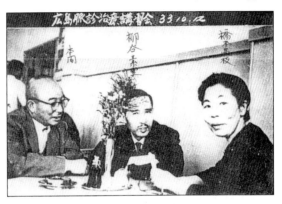

Figure 131: HONMA, YANAGIYA AND HASHIMOTO, (left to right,) the three most influential teachers and transmitters to the West of Japanese Five Element based MT.

Chinese medicine, including acupuncture, moxibustion, herbology and the other disciplines which I haven't discussed, was introduced into Japan early on. Most sources date the beginning of this transmission to the Han dynasty, but some speculate that contacts with China and its nascent medical tradition might have even preceeded the Zhou dynasty (c.1500 B.C.).[288] In any case, Japanese medicine borrowed heavily from traditional Chinese medicine

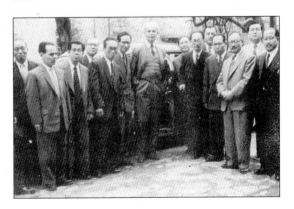

Figure 132: NOBEL LAUREATE Hans Selye visiting Yanagiya at the Tokyo School for the Blind in 1957.

until the Edo period, around 1630, when newly available European books and contacts were forbidden and Japan went into a period of isolation that likewise affected contacts with China. Thus the part of traditional

Chinese medicine which never became popular in Japan was the developments that took place in the Qing dynasty which were in turn precursors of TCM. This bit of history explains in part why TOM as practiced in Japan is so different from TCM as practiced in China, even though they share an enorous common history.

Prior to the Edo period, the major schools of medical practice in Japan[289] followed those in China, especially the four "Great Schools" of the Jin and Yuan dynasties. These included the Rishu Igaku (based on the teachings of Li Dong-yuan and Zhu Zhen-heng), and the Ryucho Igaku (based on the teachings of Liu Wan-su and Zhang Congzheng), together comprising the Gosei or school of latter-day thought. The Chinese teachings on which these schools based themselves were originally brought to Japan by Tashiro Sanki[290] (Fig.133) (1465-1537) who had studied for twelve years in China, and whose methods were popularized by his student Manase Dosan (Fig.134) (1507-1594) who in turn became famous after successfully treating the Shogun Ashikaga Yoshiteru for a serious illness.[291]

Opposed to the teachings of the Gosei school there arose a number of divergent traditions each of which developed a uniquely Japanese approach. One commonly contrasts the Gosei with the Koiho or school of ancient thought which rejected all the innovations in Chinese medicine after the *Shang Han Lun*, (*Treatise on Cold-Induced Disorders*) which it adopted as its model scripture. Its basic thrust was to return the practice of medicine to empirical observations made on real patients, and to disregard most theoretical constructs. The founder of this movement was Nagoya Gen-i (1638-1696) who originally tried to combine the strategies of each of the Four Great Chinese Schools into a common pool from which one would draw the best remedy as dictated by the empirical presentation of the patient.[292] The Koiho approach was popularized by Goto Gonzan (Fig.135) (1659-1733) who reduced all theories of pathology to a single phenomenon—the stagnation of "Original Energy" (Yuan Qi), which was differentially treated depending on where it manifested on examination. He used moxibustion extensively to activate the movement of Yuan Qi.[293] Further developing the idea of the basic identity of all forms of pathology, Yoshimasu Todo (Fig.136) (1702-1773) taught that all disease stems from one type of "poisoning" and that treatment which eliminates this poison always causes an initial worsening of the symptoms before recovery ensues.[294] This idea, which is similar to both the Hippocratic theory of "crisis" and the homeopathic "law of cure" is interestingly found in LA but not in most other contemporary approaches to acupuncture. Todo's son Yoshimasu Nangai (Fig.137) (1750-1813) is best remembered as the originator of the pathological theory of Qi, Blood and Fluids which he claimed could explain how one

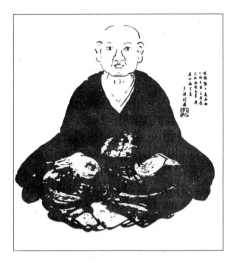

Figure 133: TASHIRO SANKI (1465–1537), who transmitted Jin-Yuan dynasty Chinese medical practices to Japan, initiating the Gosei or latter-day school.

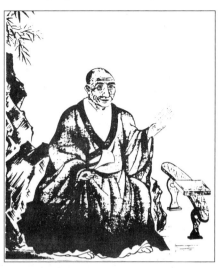

Figure 134: MANASE DOSAN (1507–1594), who became the most famous practitioner of the Gosei school after successfully treating the Shogun.

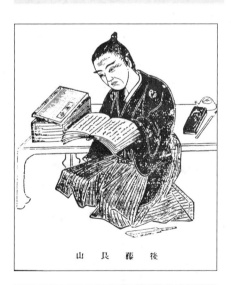

Figure 135: GOTO GONZAN (1659–1733), popularizer of the Koiho or school of ancient thought, opposed to the Gosei school. Goto also broke with the tradition whereby doctors had been shaving their heads in the manner of Buddhist priests.

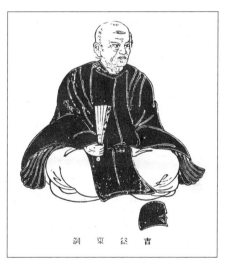

Figure 136: YOSHIMASU TODO (1702–1773) proposed that all diseses share the same pathological mechanism, a poisoning of sorts (ichidoku), and that successful treatment provokes a "healing crisis" during which the poison is eliminated.

type of poison (ichidoku) could produce such variable manifestations,[295] and this theory is still widely employed by Japanese practitioners. One consequence of the Koiho approach, which as I've said took the *Shang Han Lun* as its model, was to emphasize herbal medicine as the method for treating the root of the illness, and to relegate acupuncture to a more symptomatic adjunctive role. Thus, although in spirit the Koiho approach might seem fruitful as a source for the development of LA, in fact it rejected the whole Five Element paradigm on which LA is built.

There were however other derivatives of the Gosei school which did not subscribe to the Koiho teachings.[296] The earliest one was developed by Nagata Takuhon (Fig.138) (1513–1630) who taught that all treatment should be based on supporting the patient's "natural force," which he thought could only be done by working on the patient's feelings (or soul or mind). Nagata lived to be 118 years old, and successfully treated Shogun Hidetada, but still his tradition did not survive.[297] Another tradition which also died out was the Mubun school of Misono Isai (c. 1685) which disregarded all other aspects of Oriental medicine, focussing all attention on the diagnosis and treatment of the abdomen or Hara. The Mubun method involved tapping gold and silver needles into the abdomen with a small mallet, and although its specif-

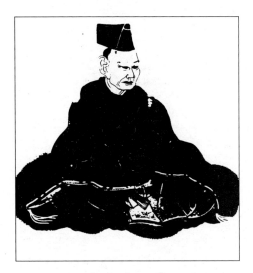

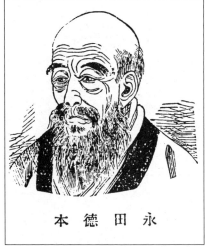

本　徳　田　永

Figure 137: YOSHIMASU NANGAI (1750–1813) developed the theory of differentiating illnesses into pathological patterns of Qi, Blood or Fluids, an approach still in vogue among some Japanese practitioners.

Figure 138: NAGATA TAKUHON (1513–1630), a vigorous proponent of the psychological, mental and spiritual approach to medical treatment, lived to 118 years of age.

ic methodology didn't survive, it was responsible for the emphasis of Japanese medicine on the Hara and abdominal diagnosis, which was adopted by all the other schools—Gosei, Koiho, and that developed by his contemporary, Sugiyama Waichi (Fig.139) (1610-1695) whom many consider to have been Japan's greatest acupuncturist of all time.

In Japan, most public (as opposed to court) acupuncturists have traditionally been blind practitioners.[298] Sugiyama, who was trained by the Emperor's physician Irie Yoshiaki, originated this tradition, which focussed on local as opposed to systemic diagnosis and treatment— palpating the body for abnormalities in texture, temperature, sensitivity, etc. He had a very inauspicious start, having been thrown out by his teacher for causing too much pain with his needling.[299] One day while walking, he tripped, and when he fell his hand grasped a straw and a pine needle by accident. He was suddenly inspired to try inserting needles through a guide tube, which method he developed to become the standard Japanese needle technique, since it lends itself to painless or almost painless insertions (Fig.140). He became a very influential acupuncturist and was appointed Grand Master by the Shogun.[300]

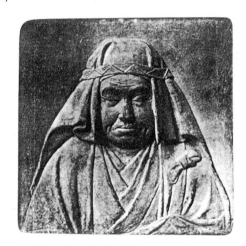

Figure 139: SUGIYAMA WAICHI (1610–1695), initiator of the tradition of training the blind as acupuncturists in Japan, he introduced many innovations into acupuncture practice.

Doctor Irie taught him that true healing was a gift of one's Spirit, and that one should not practice without this quality.[301] The blind acupuncturists who inherited Sugiyama's tradition are noted for having a "sixth sense" which is probably an expression of their spiritual development. Sugiyama introduced not only the guide tube, but also a number of extremely delicate yet sophisticated needling techniques, basing his methods on the classical teachings to be found in the *Nei Jing* and *Nan Jing*. He established 54 acupuncture schools for the blind in Tokyo which have been the training centers for the majority of Japan's acupuncturists during the last 300 years (52% of current Japanese acupuncture practitioners are blind).[302]

The final school of Japanese medicine that I should mention was called Rangaku, meaning Dutch studies. This was really a generic term for Western medicine, since the Dutch were the most privileged of

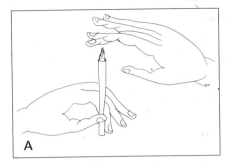
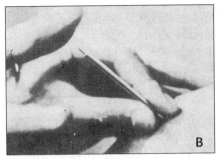

Figure 140 A and B: THE GUIDE TUBE FOR INSERTING NEEDLES, introduced by Sugiyama to facilitate painless needling. The needle handle which projects slightly past the tube is gently tapped a few times to accomplish insertion.

the Western powers in Japan during the Edo period. It was in reaction to the Westernization of acupuncture (which the Rangaku school inspired) that the Meridian Therapy movement developed, and its forerunner was a traditionalist who was greatly influenced by the Sugiyama style, Sawada Ken (Fig.141) (1877–1938). Sawada was from a samurai family, and learned acupuncture as a teenager in Kyoto, after first studying jujitsu and bone setting from a master practitioner. He spent many years developing his skills as a practitioner while living in Korea,

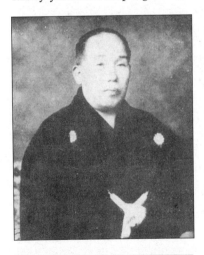

Figure 141: SAWADA KEN (1877–1938), a traditional acupuncturist of great popularity following his successful treatment of the Emperor, and one of Yanagiya's inspirations.

before returning to practice and teach in Tokyo. His style of treatment emphasized the Command Points: Five Element, Source, Alarm and Back Shu Points. Sawada was sufficiently famous to have been selected to treat the Emperor, although he was forbidden to talk or use needles—all he could do was palpate and apply moxibustion![303] In spite of these restrictions his treatments were successful and his fame spread, galvanized by the sensationalization of his results by the journalist Nakayama Tadanao in the 1920's.[304] Nakayama was an associate of both Sawada and George Ohsawa, and his book glorifying Sawada was a forerunner of the one which Ohsawa and Soulié de Morant translated into French just as acupuncture was beginning its development in

Europe. Although Sawada did not emphasize Five Element theory, he was adamant that acupuncture must be based on the classics, and it was this aspect of his teachings that was taken up by Yanagiya.

Yanagiya was the son of an acupuncturist who graduated from the first acupuncture school in Japan that was not devoted to blind practitioners. He received his acupuncturist's license at seventeen years of age, and by twenty-one he had started his own school, based on the rallying cry, "back to the classics." Yanagiya was a visionary, whose goal was "to revive the classical style of acupuncture that had been lost in antiquity."[305]

Unfortunately, although books such as the *Nei Jing* and *Nan Jing* were preserved, the practical methodology of classical acupuncture had been lost, so it had to be rediscovered—by study, meditation, self-development and experiment. Thus although the methods of Yanagiya and his school are called "classical acupuncture" there was no direct lineage of teacher to disciple from some distant "golden age." Yanagiya's personal Five Element treatment style used the four-needle technique which he learned from the Korean writings of Sa Am[306] in the 1600's, but Yanagiya encouraged his disciples, who were many (Fig.142), to find their own most effective methods, and so there are numerous variations of Five Element Japanese acupuncture. The common thread, which Yanagiya taught in the school he founded in 1927, was pulse diagnosis (myakushin) based on the *Nan Jing.* Yanagiya's approach came to be known as keiraku chiryo or Meridian Therapy (MT) which basically refers to Five Element methodology.

A particularly interesting individual, from the perspective of LA was Inoue Keiri, (Fig.143) (1903–1967), one of Yanagiya's first students. He was a Buddhist monk who initially became famous for treating all his patients with a single needle in a single Point, claiming that that was the only way to know precisely what effect each Point had.[307] There are numerous similarities between Japanese

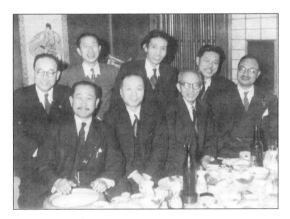

Figure 142: YANAGIYA'S DISCIPLES IN 1955. From left to right, top row: Takeyama, Tobe, Maruyama, Ishino; bottom row: Nishizawa, Honma, Inoue, Okabe. They all contributed editorial assitance to the periodical Ido No Nippon and of this group only Nishizawa and Tobe were still alive in 1993.

MT and LA as I indicated in discussing Ohsawa's text, which can now be seen as clearly derivative of this school. Additional points of similarity with LA are the following:

1) All human beings are individuals, born with characteristics that distinguish each one from the other. For every one hundred patients, therefore, there will be one hundred different symptoms requiring one hundred different types of treatment.[308]

2) People are constitutionally of 10 types, i.e., Excess or Deficient in one of the Five Elements.[309]

3) Diagnosis and treatment are aimed at the deepest level of imbalance in the Five Elements, to bring the most out of balance phase back in—essentially parallel to the causative factor (CF) of LA.

4) Diagnosis is by the five colors (on the same parts of the face as in LA), five sounds, five odors, five emotions plus the other elemental attributes—tastes, climates, fluids, exhaustions, etc... plus palpation of the pulse, abdomen and Meridians.[310]

5) Meridian palpation of the abdomen must be conducted very gently; one should hardly be able to discern whether or not one's hand is actually touching the skin.[311]

6) The Five Element diagnosis and treatment is asymptomatic. That is, the symptoms which the patient presents are not directly addressed by the treatment.[312]

7) The strengthening of Vital Energy through Fundamental Healing (root treatment) will eventually result in the removal of all the symptoms and discomforts of the patient, but certain complicated cases involving severe physical disturbances may require a long period of time to cure. Targeted Healing (i.e. symptomatic treatment) speeds up the process.[313]

8) If there is no internal weakness or injury, external causes of illness cannot affect the body. . . Therefore, rather than focussing on the Wind, Cold, Hotness, Dampness and so forth that attack from the outside, or any of the other external agents of disease (outside conditions), the Doctrine of the Causes of Illness makes the internal factors (inside conditions) of the patient the issue of central concern. Internal factors include the protective ability of the Meridians, the constitutional make-up of the individual, and abnormalities among the Seven Emotions.[314]

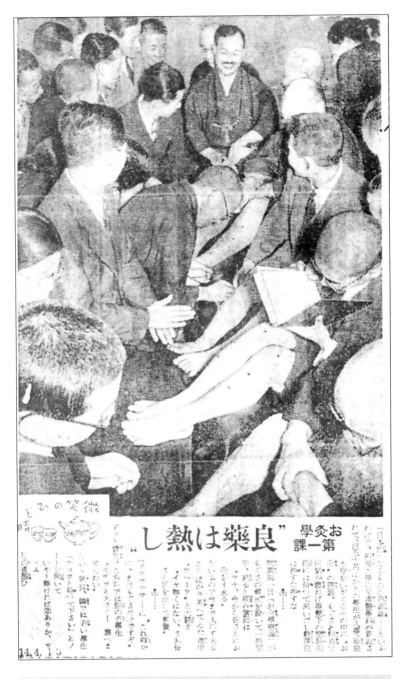

Figure 143: INOUE KEIRI (1903–1967) GIVING TREATMENT while Yanagiya looked on at Tokushoku College in 1939. Inoue together with Takeyama and Okabe coined the term Meridian Therapy (MT) to describe their common approach to treatments.

One final point I'd like to make about MT, and its similarity to LA, is that it is a consciously created style of treatment that is based on both classical doctrine and empirical testing. As Shudo Denmei (Fig.144) puts it, "It is a unique system of classical acupuncture born of the modern era."[315] The term Meridian Therapy was coined by three of Yanagiya's disciples, Takeyama Shinichiro (1900-1969), Okabe Sodo (1907-1984) and Inoue Keiri (1903-1967) who tried many methods in search of an effective treatment style consonant with the *Nan Jing*. According to Fukushima Kodo, (Fig.145) (b. 1910), these three "overcame a gap in history of more than a thousand years when they reinstated the teachings of Meridian Therapy. It was the first time in recent history that the question of akashi (conformational pattern) was revived, and acupuncture as akashi-based therapy was conducted in its true, original form."[316]

I think I've outlined enough of Japanese MT and its history to demonstrate that it was an important contributing basis for LA, and I've proposed one way in which this style was probably transmitted to Worsley. Before elaborating on that connection, we should first go back to Europe where we left Soulié de Morant and discuss the career of Dr. Roger De la Fuÿe, who learned Soulié de Morant's style of acupuncture and greatly expanded the homeopathic connection into a system he called homeosinatrie.

Roger De la Fuÿe is an intriguing figure in the history of Western acupuncture (Fig.146). Depending on your point of view, he can be seen as embodying either the best or the worst of that tradition. He was a physician whose father was the Commanding General of the French army during the time when Indochina was a French territory.[317] The custom at the time was for territorial subjects to be granted French citizenship, and thus there was a lot of interchange between the Indochinese—especially the Vietnamese—medical establishment and the French doctors—particularly through the Supreme Military Medical Academy in Paris called the Hôtel Val de Grace. De la Fuÿe had become acquainted with Soulié de Morant in 1933, and basically incorporated all of Soulié de Morant's teachings as his own, with an emphasis on the concordance between acupuncture and homeopathy. He began teaching in 1943 and published two main works; *Traité D'Acupuncture* (1947) and *L'Acupuncture Moderne Pratique* (latest edition posthumously 1972), In a 1989 article on the history of acupuncture in France, Dr. Monnier describes the first period of acupuncture in France as that of "De la Fuÿe and Soulié de Morant, one a physician and not a sinologist utilizing the material brought from the Far East by the other—a sinologist, but not a physician."[318] This tension between the roles of physician and sinologist was the first instance of much of the subsequent difficulties in the establishment of acupuncture in the West under two guises: 1) Who should be allowed to practice? Physicians, lay practitioners, both? and 2) What style of acupuncture is best? Traditional (whatever that is—but at least it means studying the classical teachings), or modern scientific, i.e., medical?

In 1945 De la Fuÿe founded the French Acupuncture Society (SFA) and in 1946 the International Acupuncture Society (SIA). In particular, the sixth SIA conference, which took place in May of 1952 in Paris, was notable for the presentation by Vietnam's Prince Buu-Loc, himself an eminant acupuncturist and educator.[319] Through his educational and organizational work, De la Fuÿe became recognized as the leading figure in French acupuncture (Fig.147), and was the main influence on the two most prominent contemporary physician-acupuncturists outside France; Johannes Bischko (Fig.148) in Austria and through him, Felix Mann (Fig.149) in England.

The first sign that De la Fuÿe's legacy was not going to be spotless was his behavior towards Soulié de Morant, his former mentor. For political reasons, in 1950, he instigated proceedings against Soulié de Morant for practicing medicine (i.e. acupuncture) without a license.[320] The charges were subsequently dropped for lack of evidence—no one would testify against Soulié de Morant—but I don't think acupuncture in Europe has yet to recover from this dastardly behavior by De la Fuÿe. If my historical narrative leaves the reader with one idea, I hope it will be that all acupuncturists should cooperate and honor their more than 2,000 years of teachers, regardless of their social status. No one has all the answers, and those that have merit will survive only if we all learn to respect one another.

Turning to the second issue—traditional versus "scientific" acupuncture, I've already indicated that De la Fuÿe was the main influence on the leaders of the "scientific" school—Drs. Bischko and Mann. Not being a student of the classics, De la Fuÿe failed to impress the traditionalists. In fact, in 1955 Yanagiya himself came to Paris for the International Acupuncture Congress as the delegated representative of the MT group in Japan (Fig.150), and an historic encounter between these two leaders occurred.[321] Yanagiya spent three months in Europe trying to understand the French (and derivative German) methods which were based more on Yin Yang thought than on the Five Elements—opposite to the approach common in Japan. He met many of the prominent European practitioners and got along with all of them except De la Fuÿe (seen in Fig.151 lecturing at the 1955 Congress, with the Japanese translator Dr. Sakaguchi interpreting for Yanagiya). Yanagiya demonstrated his style of treatment, which as shown involves a solid understanding of symptomatic treatment in addition to energetic balancing (Figs.152 A and B). The outcome was that De la Fuÿe criticized Yanagiya, among other things, for taking too much time in

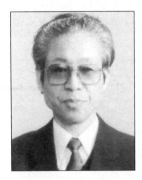

Figure 144:
SHUDO DENMEI,
author of *Introduction to Meridian Therapy,* the clearest presentation of this style of acupuncture in English.

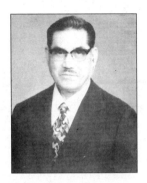

Figure 145:
FUKUSHIMA KODO,
leading proponent of MT among the blind Japanese acupuncturists, and author of *Meridian Therapy* which is the most advanced clinical text on this subject available in English.

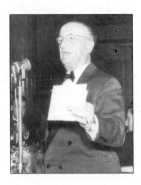

Figure 146: ROGER DE LA FUŸE (d. 1961), the political and organizational spearhead of the physician-acupuncturists in France who came after Soulié de Morant, he strove to integrate acupuncture and homeopathy into "homeo-sinatrie."

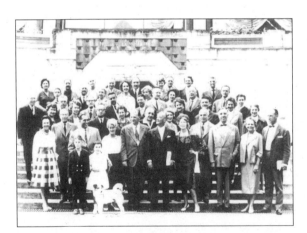

Figure 147: DE LA FUŸE
surrounded by his colleagues in the International Acupuncture Society (S.I.A.), date unknown. De la Fuÿe is in the center of the photograph, just to the left is Bischko and just above De la Fuÿe is Schatz. The photograph captures many of the luminaries of the S.I.A., but I have only identified the individuals whose work is mentioned in this text.

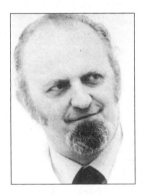

FIGURE 148:
JOHANNES BISCHKO,
Austrian disciple of De la Fuÿe and head of the Ludwig Boltzmann Acupuncture Institute in Vienna. Bischko has published numerous books and articles on acupuncture.

giving treatment, and Yanagiya responded that De la Fuÿe seemed incapable of comprehending traditional thought—not only the Five Elements, but the Dao itself which mandates that each patient be treated individually with full attention, not as materials to be treated mechanically. De la Fuÿe just got mad—actually he was aware of how unfavorably he impressed many people, but he said he just didn't care, that his legacy of organizational and educational work would justify him in the course of time.

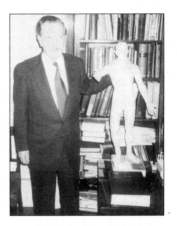

Indeed, it is through De la Fuÿe that the European acupuncture community received the teachings of Soulié de Morant, but one example might illuminate how his teachings also initiated confusion amongst European acupuncturists. In *L'Acuponcture Chinoise*, Soulié de Morant had presented the 12 Meridians in alphabetical order, which in French begins with the Heart, le Coeur, (which presentation Soulié de Morant used for didactic purposes only). He clearly indicated that the traditional ordering of the Meridian circulation starts with the Lung, and follows the Horary cycle of flow. In *Traité d'Acupuncture*, De la Fuÿe adopted Soulié de Morant's presentation of the Meridians starting with the Heart, but

Figure 149: FELIX MANN, foremost British physician-acupuncturist and founder of the British Medical Acupuncture Society, his early books championed traditional acupuncture while his later works pointedly rejected traditional theories.

incorporated this teaching into a code of Roman numerals from I through XII in the Horary sequence starting with the Heart as I! This nomenclature., and its divorce from traditional thought, but rather based on a faulty understanding of Soulié de Morant's writings, is a good example of how divisions occur amongst different groups of practitioners. I will elucidate the link which explains the transmission of this revisionist nomenclature from De la Fuÿe to Leamington shortly, but for now I simply want to explain the origin of this system of terminology which sets practitioners of LA apart from those of other styles of acupuncture.[322]

As I indicated, De la Fuÿe was the central figure in French acupuncture until his death in 1961. Outside of France, his initial influence was in Germany and Austria where his students included Doctors Bischko, Bachmann, Stiefvater and Schmidt. This linkage began in 1950 when Bachmann (Fig.153), a former military officer and the first President of the German Acupuncture Association, and Schmidt (Fig.154), the first editor of the German Acupuncture Journal, attended the S.I.A. Conference in Paris organized by De la Fuÿe. They both were physicians who had naturopathic backgrounds and were eager to learn the traditional acupuncture being taught in France. Stiefvater was more a writer than a practitioner, but is important because his 1953 German work, *Acupuncture As Neural Therapy*, along with De la Fuÿe's *Traité* was the basis for Denis Lawson-Wood's initial book in English about acupuncture, *Chinese System of Healing* written in 1959, and Stiefvater's 1955 work, *What Is Acupuncture?* was one of the first books on acupuncture to be translated into English— by Leslie Korth in 1962.

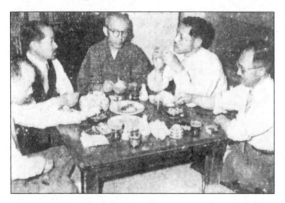

Figure 150: MT STRATEGY SESSION.
Left to right: Honma, Nishizawa, Inoue, Ishino and Yanagiya discuss their goals in sending Yanagiya to the S.I.A. Congress in France in 1955.

Heribert Schmidt, originally from Stuttgardt, died in 1995 just as this manuscript was being completed. He was a very busy and influential figure.[323] In addition to editing the German Acupuncture Journal starting in 1952, he also co-authored with De la Fuÿe the German version of *Modern Acupuncture* in 1952. Then he jumped ship, so to speak, and went off to Japan where he studied with everyone, including Yanagiya and his many associates, and brought all of the Japanese Five Element tradition back to Europe. His presentation of Soulié de Morant's tradition in Japan (Fig.155) was the basis for Yanagiya's 1955 study trip to Europe, and he was also present at Ohsawa and Hashimoto's classes in Europe in 1958. He was quite a busy fellow. Figures 156 and 157 illustrate some of his activities. He stud-

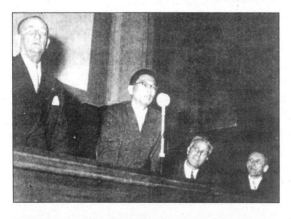

Figure 151: DE LA FUÿE, LECTURING
at the 1955 S.I.A. Congress in Paris, with translation by Dr. Sakaguchi.

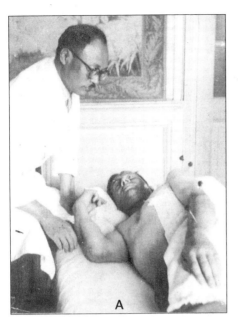

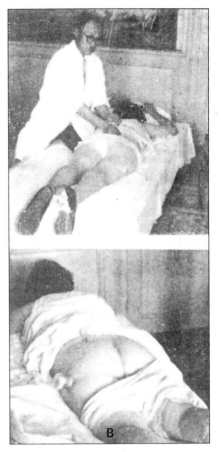

Figure 152: YANAGIYA
(A) demonstrating the use of moxa on the handle of the needle (kyutoshin) in Europe. Compare to Figures 100-102 in which the Chinese version of this technique is shown. (B) demonstrating "cupping," another traditional component of Oriental medicine with which European practitioners were relatively unfamiliar.

ied with Akabane Kobe (Fig. 158), who was close to Yanagiya, travelling with Akabane around Japan on a lecture tour, and translating his writings into German. Throughout the 1950's and 1960's, he held many workshops which introduced Japanese acupuncture in France and Germany,[324] and for a while produced a monthly newsletter with a circulation of over 100 copies. From 1951 to 1967 he was the Vice-President of the German Acupuncture Association, under Bachmann, and took over the Presidency from 1967–1971. He managed to also visit and study in Hong Kong in 1953, and received an honorary professorship from Tokushoku College in Tokyo in 1954 (Fig.159). His contributions to European acupuncture include the introduction of the Five Element methodology, with its unique style of pulse and abdominal diagnosis, the Akabane test, and some of the approaches to symptomatic treatment of the Sawada school. He translated Honma's Five Element Chart into German (Fig.160), the one I've already shown to be the basis for Worsley's version. In his later years

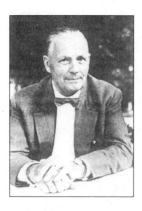

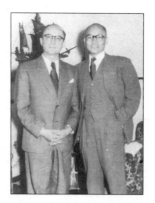

Figure 154:
HERIBERT SCHMIDT
and "colleague" in Hong Kong (the colleague to be identified in this chapter). Schmidt, originally a disciple of De la Fuÿe, subsequently studied with many teachers in Japan and Hong Kong, principally those from the MT tradition.

Figure 153:
GERHARD BACHMANN, disciple of De la Fuÿe and first President of the German Acupuncture Association.

Figure 155: SCHMIDT DEMONSTRATING
European acupuncture techniques for Yanagiya and colleagues in Tokyo in 1953. Yanagiya is just to the left of Schmidt, while above and behind Schmidt are Honma and Inoue.

(pictured below)

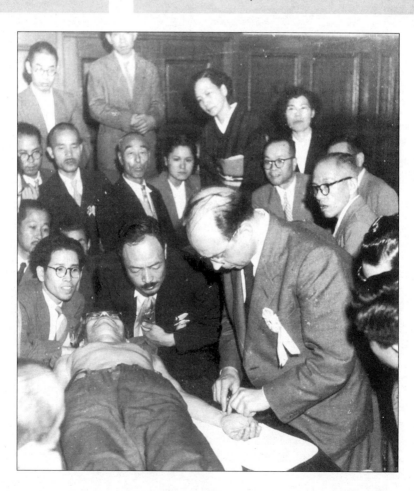

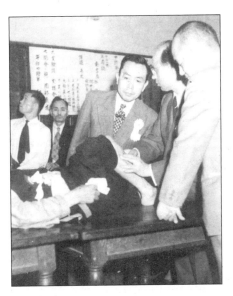

Figure 156: SCHMIDT
preparing to treat while Manaka Yoshio looks on. Schmidt's mystery colleague of Figure 154 is seen again.

(1978) he turned away from Five Element theory and developed what he called Constitutional Acupuncture, based on the teachings of the *Nei Jing* and *Shang Han Lun* as transmitted by the herbal kampo tradition which he studied under Otsuka Kaisetsu (Fig.161) (1900–1980), the acknowledged master of this tradition in Japan.

We're inching our way closer to uncovering the roots of LA, but we should first take an overall look at the origins of acupuncture in England. I've mentioned Lawson-Wood's initial publication in 1959 of De la Fuÿe's and Stiefvater's teachings. Lawson-Wood was actually commissioned by De la Fuÿe to translate his writings into English, but this project collapsed with De la Fuÿe's death in 1961.[325] In 1962, Dr. Felix Mann began publishing his series of books on acupuncture, again incorporating the Soulié de Morant–De la Fuÿe–Bischko tradition, but bolstered by his studies with the Vietnamese Dr. Van Nha in France (1958), and his own attempts to learn to read medical Chinese for access to both the

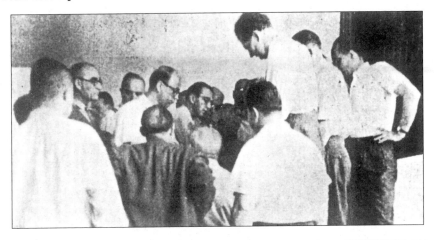

Figure 157: SCHMIDT TEACHING
Akabane's examination and treatment methods in Europe in 1955.

classical and contemporary works on acupuncture. The influence of his writings on LA can be seen most clearly in the "Function of Acupuncture Points" given in his second book, *The Treatment of Disease*

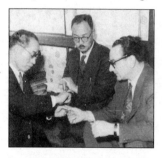

Figure 158:

AKABANE KOBE,

an associate of Yanagiya's who developed the test which bears his name and which is used in LA, is shown on the left with Yanagiya and Barat Dupond, a travelling companion of Schmidt's.

by Acupuncture (1963). This listing is derived from mainland Chinese texts written in 1959 and 1960, and interestingly has many spiritual and emotional indications not usually found in TCM writings. The Leamington course syllabus originally included this list of Point indications as the major resource for therapeutic reference. Graduates of Leamington will recognize, for example, the indications of Heart 9 for expressionless voice, Small Intestine 5 for talkativeness, Circulation-Sex 4 for fear of people and Gallbladder 39 for bad temper. These all came from this text by Felix Mann. It is also tempting to attribute a number of the other components of LA to Mann's influence: in sequential order in his first book he introduced the Law of Five Elements, the Mother-Son Law, the Husband-Wife Law, and the Midday-Midnight Law, the identical sequence and terminology used by Worsley in the title of his rendition of Honma's chart as previously shown. One must keep in mind however, that this grouping of the laws of acupuncture (which is no longer taught for the most part in TCM) is directly derived from Soulié de Morant. Mann also introduced the use of Entry and Exit Points, Window of the Sky Points, the Four Seas and the Four Needle technique—all components of LA which are easiest to account for as being

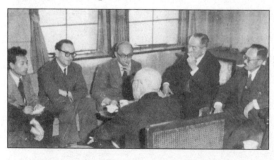

Figure 159: SCHMIDT AND DUPOND
are granted honorary professorships at Tokushoku University, while Yanagiya observes from the far right side of the picture—1954.

adoptions from Mann's first book. These aspects of traditional acupuncture can all be referenced historically, and the only one for which I have not personally seen an Oriental source is the use of the Entry-Exit Points; however, Bob Flaws has claimed that he learned the use of Entry/Exit Points from Dr. Eric Tao[326] (Fig.162), who in turn claims to have learned them in China, although he couldn't remember where—possibly from his uncle in Beijing. In a personal communication to me, Mann explained that he got that piece of information from the French literature, but he believed he had seen it in Chinese as well. In fact, the use of Entry-Exit Points is presented in *Compléments D'Acupuncture* (1955) by Jean Niboyet (Fig.163) (1913–1986), an associate of Soulié de Morant who studied intensively for a number of years with an unnamed Chinese doctor. (First a lawyer, then a doctor, then an acupuncturist, Niboyet's work was very structured, reflecting a legalistic mind.) Niboyet presents the Entry-Exit Points as part of the Zi Wu Liu Zhu style of practice used to regulate Yin and Yang, especially in terms of the Horary sequence of Meridian Qi flow. He also introduced the use of General Luo, Group Luo, Center Reunion General and Center Reunion Particular Points, information which Mann transmitted but Worsley chose not to incorporate in LA. Niboyet's approach was a combination of energetic regulation and symptomatic treatment, but based on a Yin/Yang rather than Five Element paradigm. In this context he clearly teaches the principle of "transferring" Qi from Excess to Deficient Meridians (using secondary vessels) a subject I will be examining in more detail. Finally, Niboyet should also be remembered as having

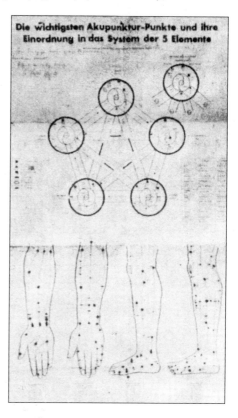

Figure 160: HONMA'S FIVE ELEMENT CHART IN GERMAN, translated by Schmidt. Compare to Figures 128 and 123.

done some of the initial work in researching the electrical properties of acupuncture Points and for trying to develop an objective method of measuring the pulses.

Returning to Felix Mann,[327] he unfortunately later recanted his initial belief in the traditional style of acupuncture, and now advocates a style of treatment based on Western medical concepts. He is also a major force behind the animosity between the medical and non-medical acupuncturists in England—the former represented by the British Medical Acupuncture Society which Mann founded. Mann's personal odyssey is a curious one, coming from a family (his mother specifically) with a strong interest in Rudolph Steiner's anthroposophical approach to medicine. He initially studied both homeopathy and herbal medicine before encountering acupuncture. In a perfect example of the Yin/Yang transformation of opposites, he has now become one of the more bitter opponents of traditional, and with it, non-physician, acupuncture. Mann, however, still takes pulses, "because it works." He charmingly describes how he chose his main teacher, Bischko, by looking for someone with the most sensitive hands, and my own personal observation is that Mann's hands are remarkably similar to Worsley's, with almost hypertrophic looking fingertips. This similarity leads me to wonder if focusing one's Qi in the digits over many years could account for such morphology.

So where were we? I was trying to set the scene for the emergence of acupuncture in England in the late '50's and early '60's.[328] Lawson-Wood's book came out in 1959, Mann's starting in 1962. At just this time, several naturopathic practitioners began attracting the attention of their colleagues because they had been studying acupuncture in Germany (from 1958–1962, principally under Bachmann) and were applying it successfully in their practices back in England. I am referring to Sidney Rose-Neil (Fig.164) and Kenneth Basham (Fig.165). They were prevailed upon by their colleagues to offer a three day seminar on acupuncture in 1962 which was attended by 68 doctors, naturopaths, osteopaths, chiropractors and physiotherapists. Leslie Korth, Denis Lawson-Wood and Nicholas Sofroniou gave short presentations at this seminar which was attended by Jack Worsley, Dick Van Buren, Malcolm Stemp and Mary Austin among others (Fig.166). Sofroniou (Fig.167) had also studied acupuncture in Germany, especially the Meridian Therapy style of Honma Shohaku, whom Dr. Heribert Schmidt had brought over from Japan. When he was asked to teach at the 1962 seminar in London, Sofroniou confined his remarks to pulse taking and Five Element theory, as these were the most coherent aspects of what he himself had learned. The seminar generated so much excitement, that there and then the British Acupuncture Association was formed, and the seeds of the British College of Acupuncture were sown. The College was originally established in Kenilworth in 1964. One can see that at its inception, the British Acupuncture Association and the College were umbrella organizations that included all the British figures I've mentioned except Felix Mann. As an interesting aside, in Figure 165 the reader may notice that Dr. Basham is seen taking his wife's pulses with his hands in the "handshake" position, and this manner of pulse-taking became the standard at the British College of Acupuncture, and

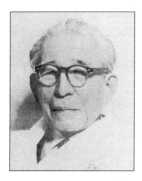

Figure 161:
OTSUKA KEISETSU
(1900–1980),
the leader of the
kampo style of herbal
medicine, another of
Schmidt's teachers.

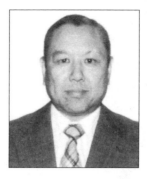

Figure 162: ERIC TAO,
a traditional acupuncture
teacher from Taiwan, now
living in Denver, was the
first acupuncture teacher of
Bob Flaws (the founder of
Blue Poppy Press which
publishes many books on
Oriental medicine) and the
translator for Worsley on his
1966 visit to Wu Wei-p'ing
(see Figure 98).

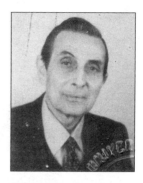

Figure 163: JEAN
NIBOYET (1913–1968),
who expanded on the
work of Soulié de Morant
by incorporating material
from an anonymous
Chinese teacher, includ-
ing the use of Entry and
Exit Points. He founded
the Mediterranean Acu-
puncture Society (S.M.A.)
in 1955.

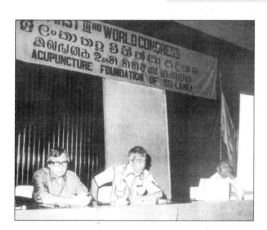

Figure 164: SIDNEY ROSE-NEIL, (center),
the first President of the British Acupuncture
Association who helped to spread the traditional teachings from Germany to the U.K.

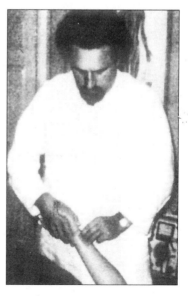

Figure 165: KENNETH BASHAM,
an osteopath who organized the
first acupuncture seminar in
England with Rose-Neil in 1962.

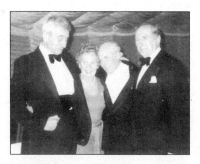

Figure 166: REUNION of attendees of the 1962 seminar at Worsley's sixty fifth birthday in 1988. From left to right: Rose-Neil, Mary Austin, Worsley and Stemp.

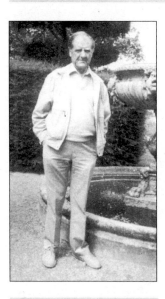

Figure 167: NICHOLAS SOFRONIOU, one of the earliest acupuncture teachers in England, is still in practice in London in 1994. He was strongly influenced by Honma, and in turn influenced Worsley, both directly and through establishing a later seminar Worsley attended at which Okabe and other Japanese practitioners taught.

later at the College in Leamington established by Worsley. The origin of this method of taking pulses is unclear—I have personally never seen anyone from the Orient use it, and Basham could not remember where he learned it, although he hypothesized that it may very well have been a reflection of his previous osteopathic training in the subtle styles of manipulative medicine which require a delicate hands-on technique. The more common style of pulse and tongue examination, typically used in TCM, is shown in Figure 168.

In the year following Rose-Neil and Basham's seminar (i.e. 1963), a group called the Naturopathic Research Association sponsored a two week course in acupuncture taught in London by the French acupuncturist, Jacques Lavier, whom I've already mentioned. Lavier's acupuncture education included several months of study in Taiwan with Wu Wei-p'ing in the 1950's but he clearly had numerous other teachers. Lavier had initially met Wu at one of the International Acupuncture conferences in Paris arranged by De la Fuÿe. Lavier's initial two week course in London was followed at a later date by a second two weeks of classes. This format is the same as that adopted by Worsley for teaching LA to his American students, so it should come as no surprise that he was in attendance at Lavier's course along with Dick Van Buren, Royston Low, Denis Lawson-Wood, Nicholas Sofroniou and others. I've already shown a picture of that class (Fig.106), and the reader might note that Lawson-Wood and Sofroniou are not in the picture. That is because they were asked to leave the class after the first week when Lavier discovered that they were already writing and teaching about acupuncture—an authoritarian approach to sharing knowledge that has unfortunately been too common in the history of acupuncture education.

Lavier, as I've indicated, was to a large degree responsible for introducing the Five Element approach in acupuncture to England,[329] where it took root the strongest, in contrast to the Rose-Neil—Basham material which had primarily reflected the Yin Yang tradition of Soulié de Morant, De la Fuÿe, and Bachmann. Unfortunately, Lavier died in 1987 leaving more or less unsolved one of the biggest mysteries concerning LA—the origin of the methodology of transferring energy via the Creative and Control cycles of the Five Elements, from Meridians in Excess to those in Deficiency, which was one of LA's central tenets from the outset. In addition to being presented at Lavier's London seminar, this methodology was also described in Lavier's rendition of Wu Wei-p'ing's writing, in a book called, *Chinese Acupuncture,* which is an annotated compendium of several of Wu's writings that was first published in English by Philip Chancellor in 1962. What's of prime interest here is that the section on the Five Elements, part 5 of the book, was not written by Wu, but by Lavier himself. Here is Lavier's own testimony: "The last section of this book is dedicated to the Law of the Five Elements, the veritable keystone of Chinese medicine. Unfortunately, my friend Dr. Wu Wei-P'ing wrote nothing on this subject. I have taken the liberty of writing this part myself, the Master having given his warm approval of the contents."[330] Figures 169 and 170 show Lavier's rendition of this material, and how reminiscent it is of Worsley's presentation. Following Lavier's introduction of this material, the Five Element transfer methodology later appeared, with minor variations, in works by Lawson-Wood (1965) (Fig.171), Mary Austin (1972) (Figs.172 and 173) and Pennell and Heuser (1973), but none of these provide any further insight into the history of this methodology. Lavier's personal history[331] casts further doubt on a Wu to Lavier lineage. Lavier began learning Chinese calligraphy at age eight when he was immobilized for four years for health reasons. His Chinese was mostly self-taught from dictionaries, and

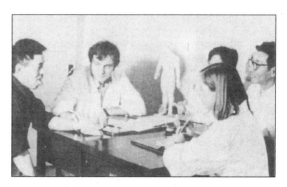

Figure 168: TCM STYLE EXAMINATION OF THE TONGUE AND PULSE.
Note the cushion which supports the patient's wrist in lieu of being held by the practitioner's free hand.

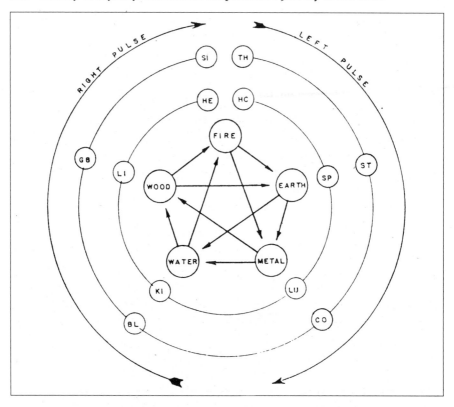

Figure 169: FIVE ELEMENT CHART PER LAVIER
from Wu Wei-p'ing's *Chinese Acupuncture*. Note the error in designating left
and right pulses which is undoubtedly a proofreader's mistake.

although he became proficient in written Chinese, specializing in the ancient forms of the characters, he never learned to speak any of the dialects, beyond a few pleasantries. Thus, it seems unlikely that he would have learned the Five Element style orally from Wu. Professionally, Lavier had originally planned to study medicine, but World War Two interrupted his training, and he instead became a dentist, serving in this capacity as a medical officer in Vietnam during World War Two when he had his first exposure to acupuncture. It was only after the War that he went to Taiwan to study acupuncture.

How then, can we account for the Five Element transfer tradition? Let's look at several hypotheses:

1. Unlikely as it may be, perhaps Lavier did indeed learn it from Wu. On the negative side, in addition to Lavier's personal contrary testimony, are many accounts of Wu's treatment style, notably by Fox, Chen and Tao among others.[332] On the positive side, in addition to

Lavier's version of Wu's book and the climate of popular belief it created, I might cite the testimony of Professor Paul Lepron, a colleague and
disciple of Lavier's who claims that the Five Element style was an oral
tradition dating back to Liu Wan-Su (1110–1200) the first of the "four
great physicians of the Jin and Yuan dynasties," who is primarily
remembered for starting the "cooling school" of internal medicine. He
is often cited by Bob Flaws for his theory of "similar transformation" to
explain the development of "evil heat" in the body. Lepron claims that
Liu Wan-su's oral tradition of Five Element acupuncture was preserved
only in Taiwan, presumably indicating Wu Wei-p'ing, but there is nothing to exclude the possibility of another unnamed Taiwanese source.[333]

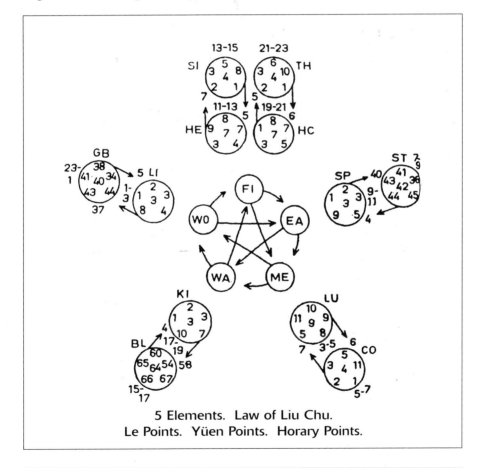

5 Elements. Law of Liu Chu.
Le Points. Yüen Points. Horary Points.

Figure 170: FIVE ELEMENT CHART PER LAVIER

from *Points of Chinese Acupuncture*, a later and more elaborate rendition that is
very close to Worsley's version. As will be discussed, Lavier claimed to have studied under Yanagiya and his disciple Nishizawa, so the similarity of his and Honma's
charts is not accidental.

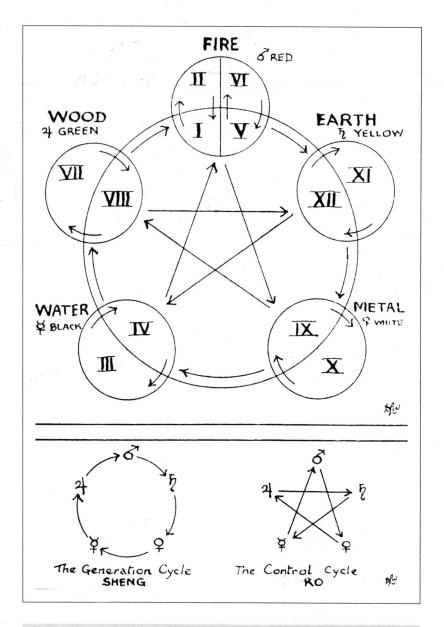

Figure 171: FIVE ELEMENT CHART PER LAWSON-WOOD,
again reflecting the influence of Japanese MT, presumably through
Sofroniou and/or Lavier.

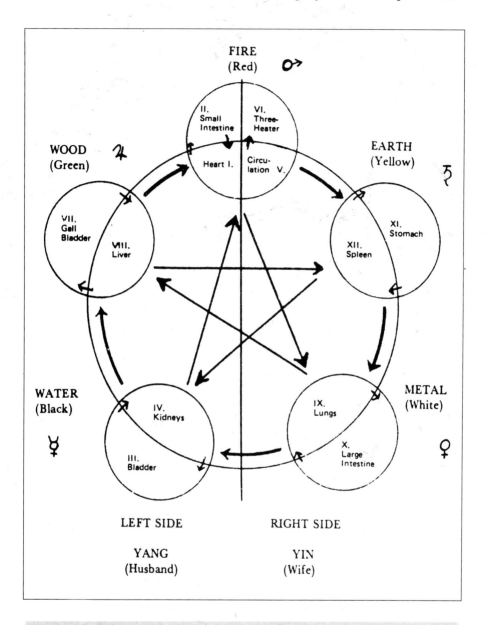

Figure 172: FIVE ELEMENT CHART PER AUSTIN,
an expanded version by Lawson-Wood which now includes the primordial
version of the Law of Husband-Wife.

Van Buren, who knew both Wu and Lavier, claims that this transmission definitely did not come from Wu, but from two other anonymous Chinese teachers, in France.[334]

Before leaving the Liu to Lavier hypothesis, I should mention that one of Lavier's other main contributions to LA is the concept of Aggressive Energy or AE, which is called just that in his lecture syllabus,[335] and whose treatment protocol calls for draining the AEP's (Back Shu Points) of the Zang Organs involved, prior to energetic balancing. The suggestion that AE is another name for Evil Qi (Xie Qi) which has transformed (similarly) into Heat, as per Liu's theory, has been correctly given already by Flaws.[336] Li Dong-yuan, during the same epoch as Liu Wan-su, recommended a similar protocol—treating the Back Shu Points of the Zang Organs for any condition resulting from the penetration of environmental Evil Qi secondary to a deficiency of central Qi.[337] He called this Yin disease (of the Zang Organs) in the Yang (the back) and attributed this approach to material presented in the *Shang Han Lun*. The symptomatology of patients with this pathology could involve sinews, bones, blood or vessels, and thus covers the gamut of presentations found with AE. A confusing issue I faced as a student of LA was Worsley's claim that if untreated, AE was invari-

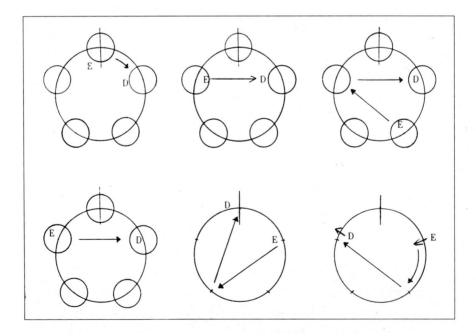

Figure 173: ENERGY TRANSFERS,
first illustrated schematically on the skeleton Five Element chart, in Austin's
Acupuncture Therapy.

ably fatal (the time to demise being inversely proportional to the num-ber of Officials "polluted" by AE). Since acupuncturists from other tra-ditions did not employ the treatment protocol specified for AE, their patients should have done worse than experience reveals. Again Lavier supplied the resolution to this dilemma in a 1966 publication[338] wherein he describes other strategies for eliminating AE, including draining it from the Five Element Command Points, which is in fact a strategy frequently employed in TCM. Thus, Lavier used the Five Element Points in two different manners: draining them in a non-transfer paradigm when AE was present, and tonifying them to transfer Righteous Qi (Zheng Qi) from Meridians in Excess to those in Deficiency only when no AE (Xie Qi) was present. In following this line of thinking then, the same Point might be drained at one treatment ses-sion, and then tonified at the next. While I'm on the subject, let me enumerate the other similarities and differences between Lavier's teach-ings and LA:

In the list of similarities, Lavier introduced the term ACI (anatomical Chinese inch) to replace Soulié de Morant's use of "pouce" (thumb) as the standard form for measurements and like Worsley, called the Horary cycle of Qi flow the Wei level of circulation. He stressed the need to palpate for Points, not merely go by anatomical landmarks or measurement. His Point locations, like Worsley's are essentially identical to Wu Wei-p'ing's. His needle technique was con-trary to Soulié de Morant's, and introduced in and out tonification, prolonged (greater than ten minute) sedation, and snatching moxibus-tion—all essential components of LA. Lavier himself felt that this dif-ference in technique was the single most important contribution to good clinical results of his style over that of Soulié de Morant. He also taught the use of Horary Points to begin the phase of energetic balanc-ing, left side tonification and right side dispersion, and seasonal pre-ventative treatment, as well as avoiding treatment during climatic dis-turbances. He also presaged Worsley's concept of the "Spirit of the Point" and presented fourteen examples of relying on Point names to validate their clinical use.[339]

As far as differences from LA are concerned, Lavier taught that symptomatic treatment was always the first approach to be used in clin-ical practice, especially for acute conditions. After the acute sympto-matic phase was resolved, the next step would be draining AE, and only after both of these were finished, would energetic balancing via Five Element pulse diagnosis be attempted—he saw this latter stage of treat-ment as essentially preventative. In spite of his focus on symptomatic treatment however, it is clear that Lavier's work was a major influence in the development of LA. He also laid the groundwork for much of the material later elaborated by the various teachers in the French

Acupuncture Association including the *Yi Jing* based energetics of Mussat (Lavier introduced the notion of inverse and contrary trigrams based on the Fu Xi order)[340] and the dialectical hierarchies of the Six Great Meridians with respect to the variable viewpoints of anatomy and physiology[341] as exemplified in the work of Kespi.[342] Finally, it should not be forgotten that Lavier pioneered the movement to base the practice of acupuncture on classical Chinese, an endeavor being carried on today by Claude Larre and his colleague Elisabeth Rochat de la Vallée of the European School of Acupuncture.

 2. A second hypothesis for the origin of the transfer methodology taught by Lavier, would be to substitute one or more alternative Taiwanese teachers for Wu Wei-p'ing as the Taiwanese source. As an alternative, Jean-Louis Blard, a French acupuncturist who knew Lavier,

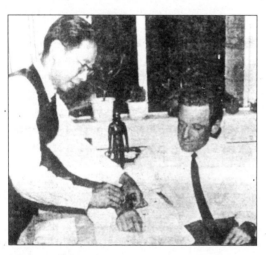

has suggested Leung Kok-yuen (Fig.174), from Hong-Kong, as the source for some of the LA information such as treating AE.[343] In my own questioning of him, Leung did not remember Lavier as one of his students, but communication was somewhat difficult as there was no translator, and the interview was therefore in English.[344] There is even testimony on this question by Lavier himself, but it unfortunately does little to resolve the confusion. In a letter to me shortly before he died, Lavier cited several teachers in Taipei, especially Chuang Yu-min (Fig.175) (1903–?) as his source for this methodology; however, Chuang's pub-

Figure 174: LEUNG KOK-YUEN, founder of the pioneering North American College of Acupuncture, is shown here treating the actor William Holden.

lished works give no hint of this methodology including numerous works available only in Chinese, and several in English such as *Chinese Acupuncture* and *The Historical Development of Acupuncture*. One would think that either of these latter two works might at least mention transfers of energy if this was an important component of Chuang's teachings.[345] Chuang was trained in the scholarly tradition of acupuncture starting at the age of fifteen,[346] first by his uncle in Jiang Su and later under a disciple of Ma Pei, a reknowned royal physician of the Qing dynasty. He emigrated to Hong Kong in 1950 and then to Taiwan in 1965, setting up a number of acupuncture schools, clinics and professional associations. It was in this context that Lavier studied with Chuang, and as they are now both deceased, we will never know the details of any transmission that may have occurred.

Another Taiwanese teacher who might have played a role in the "transfer" transmission was Eric (Hsi-yu) Tao (born in 1925). Tao emigrated from China to Taiwan in 1954 and helped Wu Wei-p'ing set up the Acupuncture Association there. Because he spoke English (learned while working for the U.S. Navy), he acted as translator for Wu when foreigners visited, including Worsley, Stemp (Fig.176), Lavier and Laville-Méry. He originally learned acupuncture from his uncle in China, and later studied with a Dr. Lee in Taiwan. He eventually moved to the U.S. where he taught material, including Five Element transfers, to Pennell and Heuser and also Bob Flaws. I interviewed him a number of times, and he was very unclear on where he had learned this methodol-

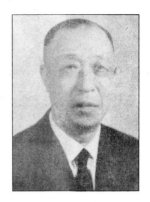

Figure 175:
CHUANG YU-MIN, · who had studied under Cheng Dan-an as related in Chapter Four, was an influential teacher in Hong Kong and Taiwan, and transmitted some of his methods to Lavier.

ogy. He thought Lavier and Laville-Méry (Fig. 177), Wu's early students, had learned mostly from old books, but he himself did not know anything about a Liu Wan-su acupuncture tradition, and had himself also been exposed to many books, Chinese as well as Japanese, that might have influenced him. (I include him in this hypothetical scheme merely to indicate that there may indeed have been a Chinese oral tradition of using the Five

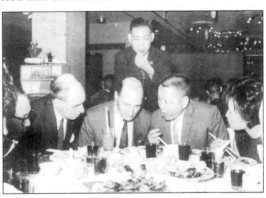

Figure 176: ERIC (HSI-YU) TAO
is seen here interpreting for Worsley and Stemp while Wu Wei-p'ing observes, at the ceremonial dinner during Worsley's visit to Taiwan in 1966.

Elements, including transfers, as Worsley teaches, but we may never see a complete account of its history and methodology.)

     3. To be rigorous in pursuing possibilities for the source of the transfer methodology, we should certainly consider Lavier's other teachers. In his 1975 text, *Vade-Mecum D'Acupuncture Symptomatique*, Lavier cited the authors of numerous books, articles and courses of study as the basis for his teachings. Two were from Taiwan (Wu Wei-p'ing and Tsui Chieh), one from Hong Kong (Chuang Yu-min), one from Beijing (Zhu Lian), one from Singapore (Wang Tchia-tchun), two from Korea (Kuon Dowon and Kim Bong Han) and three from Japan (Yanagiya Sorei, Nichizawa Michimasa and Nakatani Yoshio (Fig.178), the first two being Meridian Therapists while the third was the originator of Ryodoraku, a Five Element influenced style of electroacupuncture). As I've indicated, neither Wu nor Chuang can be verified as a putative source. Tsui (Fig.179), who published material in Chinese, was rather more Western than traditional in his orientation,[347] so he, too, can be eliminated as a possibility, as can the two Koreans. Kuon Dowon[348] (Fig.180), still practicing in Seoul, is the founder of Korean constitu-

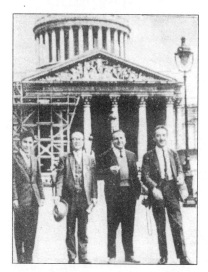

tional acupuncture, which is a Five Element based style of practice, but which uses variations of the "Four Needle Technique" for treatment as opposed to employing energy transfers. The Four Needle Technique was first described in the 1600's by a Korean monk, Sa Am, and is considered by many to be one of the high-water marks in the history of Five Element approaches to acupuncture. The Four Needle Technique is even taught as part (albeit a relatively minor one) of LA, having been described early on in the English literature by Mann.[349] Kim, on the other hand, was a North Korean researcher who had claimed to have discovered a material basis for acupuncture Points and Meridians, and whose work was widely publicized at first (Fig.181), but who later committed suicide when his findings could not be duplicated by other research workers. It is noteworthy that all of the three Japanese were teachers of Five Element styles, and so

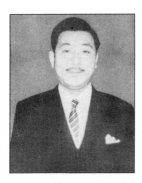

Figure 178:
NAKATANI YOSHIO,
a physician who developed Ryodoraku, a style of acupuncture that I listed in Figure 3 as mixed, being a combination of traditional and Western medical ideas and methods.

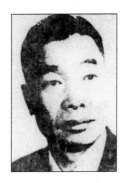

Figure 179:
TSUI CHIEH,
a Taiwanese physician who was well-trained in traditional acupuncure, tried to interpret its effects in Western medical terms.

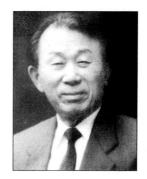

Figure 180:
KUON DOWON
is the founder of Korean Constitutional Acupuncture, which is based on an integration of the Four Constitutions herbal theory of Lee Je-ma and the Four Needle acupuncture theory of Sa Am. Kuon's methods parallel those of Yanagiya who had also based his treatments on Sa Am's Four Needle Technique.

this might be a more fruitful place to search for the origin of the transfer method. Unfortunately, most contemporary Japanese practitioners of MT that I've questioned are either unfamiliar with this method, or claim that it doesn't work![350] They use other parallel treatment protocols, and no one has identified Yanagiya or any of his students as the source of this method, so in spite of its appeal, a Japanese lineage for the energy transfers must remain an unverified and unlikely hypothesis. What Lavier may have learned from Yanagiya and Nichizawa, was the extremely delicate and gentle style of needling, which he in turn passed on to Worsley. Pennell and Heuser (who published material they had been taught about energy transfers) did however cite three other Japanese teachers whom I'll mention for the sake of completeness. Kon Kenichiro and Hosaka Rihei (both from Osaka) are unknown to me, but were described as unlikely candidates by Richard Yennie who knew them.[351] Nagayama Kunzo (Fig.182), on the other hand, deserves more serious consideration, if for no other reason than that he and Worsley visited each other's clinics and undoubtedly the two influenced each other.[352] Nagayama (1935–1991) was the director of the Kyoto Pain Control Institute, and although in his public research he frequently used electroacupuncture and various forms of symptomatic treatment, I've heard several reports that his treatment style in private practice resembled LA, using very few Points per treatment and relying very much on pulse diagnosis to identify the strongest and weakest Meridians.[353] He has unfortunately joined the growing list of participants in this story who are no longer alive to tell their tales.[354]

Being unable to confirm anyone as yet as the source of the transfer methodology, we should consider the last two of Lavier's references.

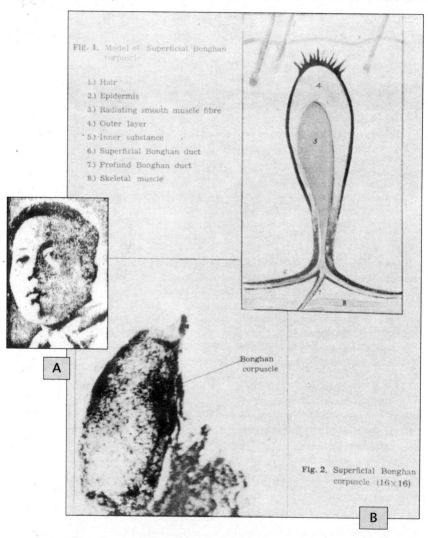

Fig. 1. Model of Superficial Bonghan corpuscle

1.) Hair
2.) Epidermis
3.) Radiating smooth muscle fibre
4.) Outer layer
5.) Inner substance
6.) Superficial Bonghan duct
7.) Profund Bonghan duct
8.) Skeletal muscle

A

Bonghan corpuscle

Fig. 2. Superficial Bonghan corpuscle (16×16)

B

Figure 181: KIM BONG HAN
(A) whose claim to have discovered an anatomical substrate for acupuncture was initially widely publiced, as in (B) from *Is Acupuncture for You?* by Worsley. His work was never corroborated and is now generally discredited.

Madame Zhu Lian (Fig.90), the reader might remember, was one of the very founders of TCM, and had a decidedly Western medical slant at that, so she can be crossed off the list. The sole remaining figure is Wang Tchia-tchunn from Singapore, whose story has proven as difficult as that of the transfers themselves, to unravel. Dr. Anton Jayasuriya (Fig.183) of Sri Lanka claims to have known him well,[355] but seems to know nothing relevant to the issue at hand other than the belief that Wang is also already deceased. Jayasuriya (born in 1930) and his students in Sri Lanka have been among the few authors to have published material on energy transfers, however these are all of a much later date than Lavier's teachings. In fact, Jayasuriya's first involvement with acupuncture seems to have been as a W.H.O. Fellow in Beijing in 1974,[356] thus his Five Element teachings are more likely to be ultimately derived from those of Lavier rather than vice-versa. There is, however, another Dr. Wang from Singapore who taught acupuncture to Westerners

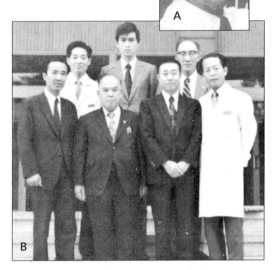

Figure 182: NAGAYAMA KUNZO A & B (front row, second from the right) with other Japanese acupuncturists including Dr. Akashi (front row, second from the left), the President of the Kyoto Acupuncture Association. The late Dr. Nagayama (M.D., Ph.D.) was the Director of the Kyoto Pain Control Institute, whose Journal listed J.R. Worsley as a member of its advisory board, along with S. Rose-Neil, R. Pennell, G. Heuser, R. Yennie and N. Van Nghi. Nagayama, as a colleague of Worsley, may have influenced the latter's understanding of the Japanese Five Element acupuncture tradition.

under the name Ed or E.C. Wong,[357] who may or may not have been the same individual as Wang Tchia-tchunn. Adding to the confusion is that this Dr. Ed Wong (Fig.184) was one of the ten sources cited by Pennell and Heuser for their information on transfers, so he must be considered as a serious candidate, being possibly linked to both Lavier and Pennell and Heuser who may have independently learned the transfer methodology from him. Ed Wong was well remembered by Eric Tao, Pedro Chan and Richard Yennie, who noted that Wong had even organized an international acupuncture conference in Las Vegas in the 1960's or 1970's which was attended by famous practitioners from both the Orient and the West, so it is even possible that he had some contact with Worsley, although that is pure speculation. It is on record, however, that Worsley claimed to have studied acupuncture in Singapore early in his career![(358)] As long as Worsley is still alive, there is some hope that this confused tangle can yet be straightened out.[(359)]

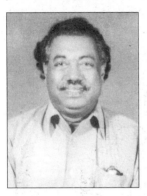

Figure 183:
ANTON JAYASURIYA, Chairman of Medicina Alternativa International, has written over 35 books on acupuncture and related subjects, since studying in China in 1974.

In regard to Ed Wong, there is an interesting conclusion to my research on the history of energy transfer lineages. Just as this book was undergoing its final revision in 1995, I obtained copies of two of the teaching manuals and a promotional brochure written by Ed Wong, which are listed in the bibliography. Almost half of the first manual (undated) is a verbatim reproduction of the therapeutic repertory (Part Four) from Wu Wei-P'ing's *Chinese Acupuncture* translated by Lavier, indicating that Wu, Wong and Lavier shared a common core of knowledge. The second manual (also undated) is perhaps of more interest in that it gives explicit instructions for transfers of energy via both the Creative and Control cycles, the latter going from Yin Organ to Yang Organ and vice-versa, thereby conforming to the teachings of Lavier, Wu, and Pennell and Heuser, while differing in this aspect only, from the teaching of Worsley. One conclusion seems obvious: Lavier, Wu and Wong shared an earlier version of the transfer dogma that Wong subsequently transmitted to Pennell and Heuser. A later version of the transfer dogma (Yin Organ to Yin Organ across the Control cycle) was in turn derived from the teachings of this group (most likely via a garbled interpretation of Lavier's teachings) and promulgated by Lawson-Wood, Austin and Worsley, whose clinical experience verified the practical utility of this alternate methodology, regardless of its lineage. The association of Lavier and Wong with the earlier version of the transfer dogma provides suggestive evidence that Wong (as Wang) was Lavier's source in this regard. Wong claimed to have been a sixth generation practitioner of acupuncture, tracing his lineage back to Wong Ham Chai, the imperial palace physician who in 1836 established the Tai I Acupuncture College in Fujian province. Wong also studied at Cheungsan Medical School in Canton as well as at other institutions in

China, Japan and Europe. He associated with many of the teachers mentioned in this chapter as illustrated in Figure 184. Eric Tao first met Wong in the late 1950's or early 1960's when Wong was living in Singapore. The timing of this scenario gives strong support to the identification of Wong as the teacher from Singapore cited by Lavier, which in turn favors the hypothesis that the transfer methodology was first taught to Westerners by Wong—Lavier being one of his earliest students. This hypothesis begs the question of whether Wong's teachings were based on a Chinese oral (family) tradition, a Chinese academic tradition or equally plausably, a Japanese tradition to which he was exposed. As Wong is no longer available, it is quite possible that this remaining bit of mystery may never be resolved.

Having mentioned Sri Lanka, there is one more teacher to include in this survey, and that is Ms. Radha Thambirajah (Fig.185), the first practitioner to establish an acupuncture practice in that country.[360] Thambirajah did not learn her acupuncture in Sri Lanka, however, but in China during the Cultural Revolution. What's interesting is that she claims to have learned there the concepts and methodologies of energy transfers via the Five Elements which she has since taught widely and still uses in her practice in

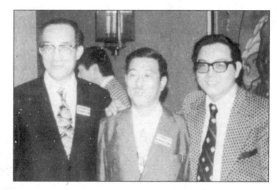

Figure 184 A (top): ED WONG (right) with Nakatani (middle) and Sakamura (left) of the Japanese Ryodoraku Society. The author's research favors Wong as the most likely Oriental transmittor of the Five Element transfer technique to the West, where it became a central component of LA dogma.

Figure 184 B (bottom): This photograph from a 1972 seminar in Kyoto, Japan organized by Ed Wong (bottom shot, right of center) for Western students shows Manaka Yoshio (top shot, third from left) as one of his teaching colleagues.

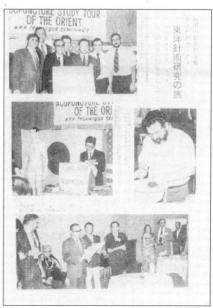

England, where she currently resides. Although it would seem almost beyond belief that the only Oriental textual source for this mysterious methodology should be found in the China of the ultra-materialist Cultural Revolution, which was the epitome of anti-traditionalism, the explanation is that she studied from 1964 to 1970 at the Shanghai Military Medical College, and the military was the only part of Chinese society to have been relatively free from the political repression going on everywhere else. The transfer methodology, as well as the use of Entry and Exit Points, another important component of LA, were both taught by her teachers (one of whom was 73 at the time) and expounded in some old texts which she reputedly still has in her possession.[361]

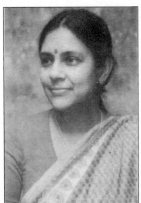

Figure 185:
RADHA THAMBIRAJAH, Sri Lankan practitioner who learned acupuncture in China during the Cultural Revolution, and who has since taught many doctrines that are not presently included in TCM.

4. Although I don't believe it, I feel that I should at least mention the possibility that Lavier himself might have devised the transfer methodology in an attempt to reconcile the teachings from his various sources. The idea of transferring Qi from locations of Excess to those that are Deficient is implied in several places in the classics, in the French texts of Soulié de Morant, and more explicitly in those of Niboyet (1951 and 1955) who explained transfers from Yin to Yang and vice-versa on the basis of activating secondary vessels. It is not impossible that Lavier adapted this thinking to a Five Element model, but again there is no real evidence. All I can say is that I have as yet been unable to find definitive references to this method prior to Lavier in 1962 and nothing that so far conclusively proves its Oriental origin. It is, of course strange that Lavier never clearly identified his sources, but possibly they had requested anonymity. I was actually told (by an official of the BAA, originally from China) that much of Lavier's translational work which purports Chinese authorship, was actually originally ghost-written by a mainland Chinese doctor who needed anonymity, so this speculation is quite plausible.[362]

Lavier was one of a a group of French acupuncturists, who not being physicians, were outside the orthodox organizations started by Drs. De la Fuÿe and Niboyet.[363] This small group, however, played an important role in bringing further acupuncture teachings from the Orient to Europe. The role of Worsley in this context is unclear. He was reported to have had extensive contact with Lavier in France[364] and two of Lavier's students, both Faubert and Laville-Méry were said to be graduates of Leamington.[(365)] Faubert, along with his colleague Laville-Méry, studied extensively with Leung Kok-yuen in Hong Kong, bringing over the teachings which Leung later incorporated into the North American College of Acupuncture (e.g., the use of near, middle and far points) when he moved to Vancouver. Faubert, who is still alive, has written a number of books in French about his teachers' methods, while Laville-Méry and his associate Dr. André Duron (Fig.186) (both deceased) both had contact with Yanagiya's group in Japan, and in fact it was the intention of the Japanese MT group to assist them in starting a classical acupuncture school in France under Dr. Duron, but the main proponents, Yanagiya, Honma and Duron all died before this could be accomplished[(366)] (Fig.187). Meanwhile, another colleague of Worsley's, Oscar Wexu (Fig.188), who was the last disciple to have been trained by Soulié de Morant,[(367)] was very active both in promoting acupuncture, and in insisting on the right of properly trained non-physicians to practice this ancient healing art. He established an acupuncture school in Montreal, where Mark Seem, a prominent American teacher and author received his training in acupuncture. Wexu was instrumental in working with teachers throughout the world to try to foster a cooperative spirit (Fig.189). For a brief time this endeavor seemed to be successful, as Wexu worked closely wih several physician-acupuncturists (Fig.190) including a president of the S.I.A., Dr. Jean Schatz (Fig.191) and one of the guiding lights of A.F.A., Dr. Nguyen Van Nghi (Fig.192). Unfortunately, coincident with Wexu's failing

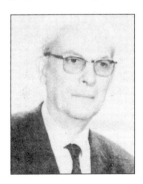

Figure 186:
ANDRÉ DURON,
French physician whose plan to open an MT oriented acupuncture school ended with the untimely demise of all the major participants.

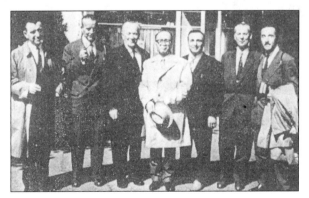

Figure 187: HONMA,
LAVILLE-MÉRY AND DURON
(fourth, fifth and sixth from the left) in 1962 while Honma was visiting Europe.

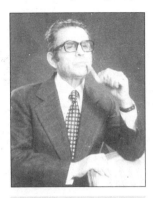

Figure 188: OSCAR WEXU, former President of the Québec Acupuncture Association and Vice-President of the S.I.A., he was the last of Soulié de Morant's many disciples.

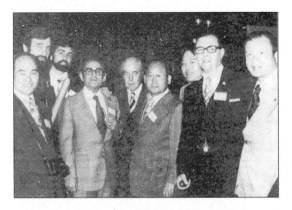

Figure 189: WEXU as first President of the International Organization of Acupuncture Associations in 1978. From left to right starting with the second individual: Rose-Neil, Mario Wexu (Oscar's son), Oscar Wexu, Worsley and Lee Chang-Bin.

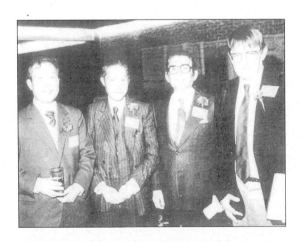

Figure 190:
FOUNDERS OF THE INTERNATIONAL ASSOCIATION OF TRADITIONAL CHINESE MEDICINE
in 1980, left to right: Xue Chongcheng, Van Nghi, Wexu and Schatz.

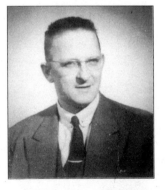

Figure 191: JEAN SCHATZ, French physician-acupuncturist who was President of the S.I.A. at the time of his demise in 1984. He counted among his teachers Soulié de Morant, Duron, Niboyet, Laville-Méry, Lavier, Nishizawa, Yanagiya, Okabe, Leung Kok-Yuen and Wu Wei-p'ing, thus epitomizing the syncretic tendencies of many European acupuncturists.

health, the rift between physician and lay acupuncturists widened again over time. Dr. Schatz is now deceased, leaving the European School of Acupuncture in the hands of his gifted collaborator, Father Claude Larre (Fig.193), who almost single handedly has trained many of today's teachers in an elementary understanding of classical Chinese—enough to begin to appreciate the classical medical texts.

The more well-known group of French acupuncturists were the physicians who carried on De la Fuÿe's initial organizational efforts, especially after his death in 1961. Starting in 1954, one of De la Fuÿe's students, a French naval doctor (continuing De la Fuÿe's and Lavier's military influence) who had recently spent several months in the Orient and became passionate about its traditional medicine, began to publish translations of Chinese medical works by a Vietnamese—this team was composed of Dr. Albert Chamfrault (Fig.194) and M. Ung Kan Sam. By 1966 Chamfrault had risen to become President of the French Acupuncture Association, and he succeeded in gathering all the physician-acupuncturists—followers of De la Fuÿe, Niboyet and others—under the same umbrella.[368] He had only just begun collaborating with Dr. Nguyen Van Nghi, a French physician of Vietnamese background, when he himself died in 1969. Dr. Van Nghi inherited the mantle, and continued to publish prolifically. His brother was the director of the Institute of Traditional Medicine in Hanoi,[369] and through him, Van Nghi had access to the North Vietnamese teaching text *Trung Y Hoc* (*Studies of Chinese Medicine*) and teaching materials from Beijing and Nanjing, which explain the strong TCM flavor of much of his (especially later) writing. On the one hand, he introduced the notion of the separate circulatory paths of Wei, Ying and Yuan Qi, emphasizing the secondary vessels, while on the other hand he also introduced the terminology of 8 Principles, 6 Stages, 4 Levels and 3 Heaters, which is the language of the "herbalized acupuncture" of TCM. Both of these contributions were incorporated, after translation from the French, into the syllabus of the British College of Acupuncture by Keith Lamont, Roy Low and colleagues, leading to a clearer divergence from LA which was untouched by this group of teachings. Van Buren reported that the material relating to the secondary vessels was a prominent teaching of Lok Yee-Kung in Hong Kong who originally came from Shanghai. As Van Nghi and Lok had definite contact,[370] Van Buren thought it more likely that this material came to

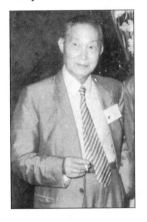

Figure 192:
NGUYEN VAN NGHI, French physician-acupuncturist of Vietnamese extraction who began to integrate both TCM and material on the Secondary Vessels into European acupuncture.

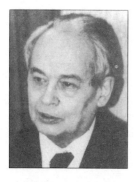

Figure 193:
CLAUDE LARRE,
Jesuit sinologist who co-founded the European School of Acupuncture (E.E.A.) with Schatz. He is well-known for his insistance that traditional practitioners study the classics in their original Chinese, so as to absorb their spirit as well as their content.

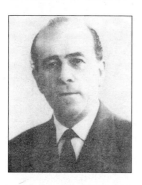

Figure 194: ALBERT CHAMFRAULT, French physician-acupuncturist who broadened De la Fuÿe's organizational efforts to also include followers of Niboyet and other disparate groups of physicians. In addition he was instrumental in promoting translations of classical texts into French, and enlarging the scope of traditional theory in the West, especially in his collaborative work with Van Nghi.

Van Nghi from Shanghai via Lok, than from Vietnam. In any case, material on the Secondary Vessels can be found in the classical medical texts such as the *Da Cheng*, but its original description along with much LA-style material can actually be found in parts of the *Dao Zang*, the "Bible" of the Daoist church which includes many combined medical/spiritual texts such as *The Yellow Court Classic*, a text that expounds the "Spirit of the Points" tradition of an energetic iconography of the body, a teaching which is fundamental to LA.[371]

I should back up for a moment and explain the origin of the different acupuncture schools in England. I already indicated that the first College of Acupuncture was an inclusive institution founded in Kenilworth in 1964. In 1969, the British College of Acupuncture under Sidney Rose-Neil and the BAA moved to London, while Professor Worsley started a separate College of Chinese Acupuncture (U.K.) in 1966 (Figs.195 and 196) which moved from Kenilworth to Oxford to Leamington Spa, where it is now located. Its graduates formed the TAS. A third school, the International College of Oriental Medicine (ICOM) was founded in 1972, when Professor Van Buren, who had previously been teaching with Worsley, started his own school in East Grinstead. This College emphasizes biorhythmic acupuncture based on Korean sources which influenced Van Buren.[372] Finally, a fourth group was started by Giovanni Maciocia (Fig.197) and other students of Van Buren, who had trained intensively in TCM in Nanjing, and founded the Register of TCM in 1979 to promote that style of acupuncture.[373] All four associations began to cooperate in 1987 under the auspices of the Council for Acupuncture, so as to present a more powerful voice for this approach to complementary medicine.

Well, now that I'm coming to the end of my story, the reader has probably realized that I never did explain how LA came to have the unique Japanese Five Element dynamic that distinguishes it from what is taught at the other British colleges. I also haven't accounted for Worsley's mysterious teachers. We know a German doctor was involved, and in addition, a Chinese teacher named Hsu and a Japanese teacher named Ono. The astute reader will have identified two possibilities for the German doctor: either Elza Munster from Hamburg or Heribert Schmidt from Stuttgardt, both deceased. They both were personally known to Worsley and I would assume both contributed to his knowledge of acupuncture. Let me return

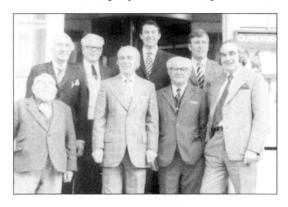

Figure 195: FACULTY OF THE COLLEGE OF CHINESE ACUPUNCTURE (U.K.)

in the early 1970's, left to right: Les Skingly, Jimmy Morgan, Harry Cadman, Jack Worsley, Tony Powell, Paul Bird, Ron Wray and Geoff Foulkes. (In his early years of teaching, Worsley was known by his first name Jack; later he consistently referred to himself as J. R. Worsley).

the focus for the moment to the man who introduced the Akabane test to Europe,[374] who was with Hashimoto and Ohsawa at their classes in Europe (where my research began) and who was perhaps the earliest of Yanagiya's European students: Dr. Heribert Schmidt. As indicated, he went to study in Japan and Hong Kong as early as 1953, and whom should he meet there, but a Chinese acupuncturist named Hsu (Fig.198)!

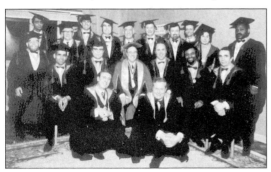

Hsu Mifoo[375] was born in Hangchow, China in 1903, and became a successful banker in Shanghai prior to World War Two. After the war, he emigrated to Hong Kong and studied at the Acupuncture Institute there for two years, from 1948–1950, chang-

FIGURE 196: COLLEGE OF CHINESE ACUPUNCTURE (U.K.) GRADUATION CEREMONY IN 1971.

Left to right, front row: Ron Wray, Dick Van Buren; middle row: Les Skingley followed by unidentified individuals except Jack Worsley in the center; rear row: unidentified individual, Paul Bird, Tony Powell, Geoff Foulkes, Jimmy Morgan, Tony Evans, and the rest unidentified.

ing careers in midlife as had many of the people I've mentioned in this narrative. Not being satisfied with the training offered at the Institute, he went to Japan where he studied and taught at several schools associated with Yanagiya's group in Tokyo (Fig.199). He had already formed

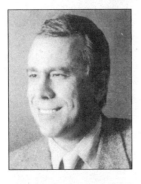

a relationship with Yanagiya (1952) prior to Schmidt's arrival in Japan (Fig.200), and undoubtedly introduced some Chinese acupuncture techniques to the Japanese (Fig.201). When Schmidt arrived, the two became good friends (Fig.202), and Hsu was invited to Germany where he became an Honorary Member of the German Oriental Medical Acupuncture Association in 1959. Remember, it was in Germany that Worsley situated his study with Masters Hsu and Ono. According to several anecdotes I have gathered from friends and family, Hsu was an extremely talented acupuncturist who typically employed only one or two needles per treatment, and who used facial color around the eyes, nose and lips as one of his most important diagnostic indicators. This description would certainly be consistent with identifying him as the teacher named by Worsley. The only concrete information Worsley ever mentioned about his "Master Hsu," outside of the fact that he met him intermittently in Germany, was that Hsu was the source of the seven dragons for seven devils treatment for "possession," which derived from the inclusion of demonology as one of the classical aspects of traditional acupuncture in China—this from a personal communication to me by Worsley. Although Worsley has claimed that his teachers uniformly practiced the identical style of treatment he teaches, I think this must be taken less than

Figure 197:
GIOVANNI MACIOCIA, one of the founders of the Register of TCM, and a leading author and teacher of TCM acupuncture and herbal medicine.

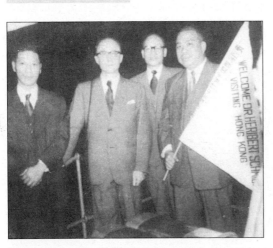

Figure 198: HSU MIFOO WELCOMES HERIBERT SCHMIDT TO HONG KONG IN 1953. Hsu is third from the left, while Schmidt is second from the left. Hsu also is the mystery colleague with Schmidt in Figure 154, and is the figure on the far right in Figure 156.

literally, as you can see in Figure 203 where Hsu is clearly taking pulses in a way that varies from that taught in Leamington. I might point
out here that the late Dr. Manaka Yoshio (1911–1989) frequently
appeared with this cast of characters, acting as a German translator
for Schmidt (Fig.204). Dr. Manaka was a unique individual who had
good relationships with many of the different Japanese schools of
acupuncture, but never became identified with any one. He did have
an important role in transmitting knowledge to the West, due to his
fluency in German and English, his collaboration with Ian Urquhart
on *The Layman's Guide to Acupuncture*, and his numerous teaching trips
to Europe and America. We see him in Figure 205 teaching blind English
massage therapists in 1984.

Master Hsu emigrated to the U.S. in 1961 and became a member of the Oregon Acupuncture Board. He also collaborated on
research projects, studying acupuncture at the Department of
Anaesthesia of the University of Washington under the supervision of
Dr. John Bonica, an international authority on pain. At the time of
his death in 1978, he had in his possession the draft of an acupuncture Point teaching manual in English, and it is interesting that the
Point names, locations and needle/moxa guidelines as well as one set
of indications are copied verbatim from Wu Wei-ping's book, while a
second set of indications are copied verbatim from Felix Mann. This is
identical to the teaching guides originally used in LA! The only difference is that in addition, Hsu also included Nakatani's Ryodoraku
Point information, betraying his interest in the Western "scientific"
study of acupuncture. In his own clinical work in the U.S., he used
electrical diagnosis in addition to the more traditional methods, and
he felt that this helped him narrow down the choice of Point to be
treated to the exact one, and to find its precise location. He was a very
broad-minded individual, and was respected by all who knew him. It
would be instructive to have access to more information about his
methods, and he apparently did write at least one article in German
which I haven't been able to locate, but most likely it will turn up in
the German Acupuncture Journal edited by Schmidt.

There are, however, several problems with definitively identifying Hsu Mifoo as Worsley's Chinese teacher. In an interview with
Malcolm Stemp in 1994, I elicited the only corraboration of there
being a Master Hsu, whom Stemp claimed Worsley met one evening
in Taiwan during their 1966 trip to the Orient. Stemp was not present
at the actual meeting due to illness, but claimed that Worsley
returned from the meeting in an exuberant state of mind saying "I've
finally seen how it all fits together." Now Hsu Mifoo lived in Hong
Kong rather than Taiwan, and subsequent research turned up a Report
in the May, 1967 issue of *The Acupuncturist* (Vol. 1, No. 1) by Worsley

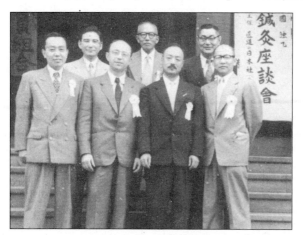

FIGURE 199: MANAKA, SCHMIDT, YANAGIYA & HSU (front row, left to right). Hsu is the only Chinese practitioner to be commonly seen with the Japanese leaders of MT, which explains one route for the reintroduction of a Five Element emphasis into the Chinese teachings which were subsequently transmitted to the West.

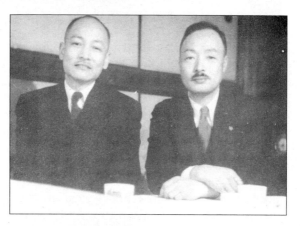

Figure 200: (above) HSU AND YANAGIYA IN 1952.

Although Hsu began sudying in Japan in 1950, from 1952 onwards he both studied and taught at Tokushoku College in Tokyo, the institution associated with Yanagiya which later granted Schmidt an honorary professorship (Figure 159).

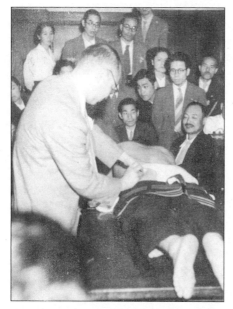

Figure 201: HSU DEMONSTRATING HIS TECHNIQUE IN JAPAN.

Yanagiya is observing, seated on the far right.

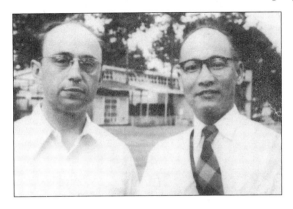

Figure 202: SCHMIDT VISITING HSU, outside the latter's residence in Hong Kong.

Figure 203:
HSU PALPATING THE PULSE.
He is feeling the pulses on the patient's right wrist with his own right hand, whereas in LA as in MT the opposite hand is always used, with the palpating fingers arching over the patient's wrist from the dorsal side. Hsu's examination is not a casual one, as evidenced by the concentration of Hsu, Yanagiya (above Hsu's hands), Honma (above Hsu's neck) and Inoue (behind Hsu's back). The venue was the Japanese, German and Chinese International Acupuncture Conference in Tokyo in 1953, where instruction in techniques from these three countries were mutually exchanged.

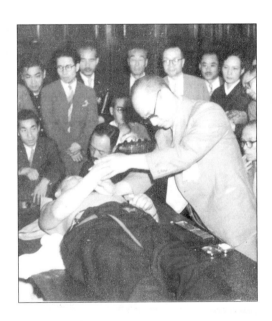

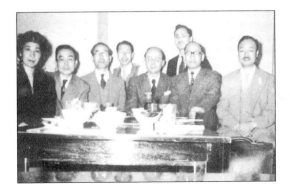

Figure 204: DINNER PARTY IN TOKYO, 1953.
Left to right: Mrs. Manaka, Manaka Yoshio, Akabane, Tobe, Schmidt, Shimizu, Hsu and Yanagiya. See also Figures 156 and 199 for other examples of Manaka's close relationship to Hsu, Schmidt and Yanagiya.

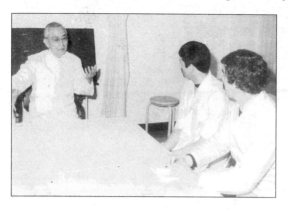

Figure 205: MANAKA YOSHIO

continuing the tradition of training the blind as therapists. He is seen here instructing two blind English massage therapists.

that two Chinese teachers had been elected to the faculty of the British College of Acupuncture, of which he was Chairman of the Board of Governors. The first was Dr. Lok Yee-Kung and the second was Dr. Hsiu Yan-Chai. Additionally, in the October, 1966 issue of *The Acupuncture Association Newsletter,* Worsley mentioned having had talks with Drs. Wu Wei-p'ing, Lok Yee-kung and Siu during his 1966 China trip. Thus, it would appear that Worsley's Chinese teacher was more likely to have been Hsiu Yan-chai. Now it turns out that there was a prominent teacher of acupuncture named Hsiu Yang-chai in Taiwan, who unfortunately died in 1993[376] (Fig.206) and this same Hsiu Yang-chai was actually present at the dinner for Worsley and Stemp in Taiwan in 1966 (Fig.207)! Eric Tao described his methods as very classical and involving the concepts of energy transfer and regulation, although not specifically Five Element in orientation. Hsiu had two main Chinese disciples,

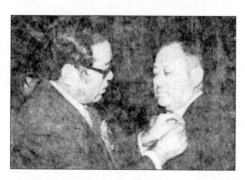

Figure 206: WU WEI-P'ING AND HSIU YANG-CHAI.

(left to right). Hsiu was on the faculty of the Acupuncture Research Institute of Taipei established by Tsui Chieh (see Figure 179) in 1950, which hosted visits by numerous foreign acupuncturists and physicians.

one of whom now lives in Denver, Dr. Frank Sun. Surprisingly, Dr. Sun was sure that Dr. Hsiu did not travel to any acupuncture conferences in Europe in the 1960's or 1970's, that he did not emphasize Five Element Theory very much, although he used it, and that he had no English students.[377] Thus we are left with yet another dilemma—Dr. Hsiu Yang-chai did live in Taiwan, where Worsley initially met him in 1966 (the time and place Stemp related Worsley meeting his Master Hsiu), but didn't travel to Europe. Dr. Hsu

Mifoo didn't live in Taiwan, but did travel to Germany (where Worsley says he studied with his Master Hsiue) where he was a member of their Acupuncture Association, and also used exactly the same teaching guides as Worsley! In addition, he was closely connected with the group of Japanese acupuncturists and with Dr. Schmidt, whose teachings somehow became incorporated into LA. The only explanation I can think of, is that Worsley knew both Hsiu Yang-chai and Hsu Mifoo and conflated them in references to his "Master Hsiue." It would appear that both teachers had a profound influence on Worsley.[378]

The final piece of the puzzle is the identity of Worsley's Japanese teacher, Ono. Thankfully, his identity appears to be unambiguous. According to Shudo Denmei (see Fig.143), the author of the first detailed book in English to describe the development of the Five Element tradition in Japan started by Yanagiya, there was only one Ono who was at all prominent in Japanese acupuncture, Ono Bunkei (Fig.208), and in fact, Bunkei Ono, the Western way of writ-

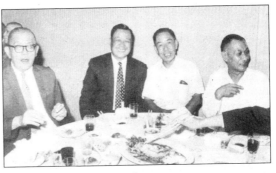

Figure 207: HSIU YANG-CHAI (second from left) at the Taiwan dinner for Worsley and Stemp in 1966. The inidividual on the far right is Chang Kwai-fu, President of the Acupuncture Association of Taichung, Taiwan. By comparing this photograph with that in Figure 97 from the same series, Hsu can be identified as the individual standing on the far right edge observing "the bow."

ing his name, is listed as a Patron of Worsley's College of Chinese Acupuncture (UK) in the undated second edition of *The Case for Acupuncture*, an out of print pamphlet listing J.R. Worsley and M.H. Stemp as co-authors. Shudo knows Ono Bunkei very well because they were neighbors, more or less, both living in Ohita prefecture. He told me the following story about Ono:[379] Originally Ono was a railroad engineer (the same profession I believe as Worsley's father), but was injured in an accident and lost a leg. He then attended one of the acupuncture schools for the blind, and began a second career. At some later time, an incident occurred in which one of his patients died, although I didn't get the details of what happened. Ono was deeply affected by it, and became almost pathologically cautious in his practice—to the point of not even inserting needles through the skin—only pressing the needles on the Points, and he discovered that for him, this worked just as well as actually inserting the needles. The non-inserted needle technique is taught by several schools in Japan, especially by Fukushima (see Fig.144), whom I've quoted previously. It was only after this episode that Ono first met and began to study with Yanagiya, and to develop his own style of Five Element MT. A similar description of Ono Bunkei's technique was related to me by Miki Shima,[380] an eclectic teacher and practitioner of Japanese styles of of acupuncture who was himself treated by Ono in 1983. He recalled that Ono used only one or two needles ("perhaps one silver and one gold") on a succession of Points which he stimulated so delicately that it felt more like tickling than needling. This "treatment" was preceeded by a lengthy (more than

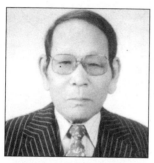

Figure 208: ONO BUNKEI, founder of Tohokai, an acupuncture association devoted to Ono's style of Five Element MT.

one hour) period of questioning and examination and was in turn followed by advice concerning different aspects of personal behavior and how it related to one's psychological state. (Interestingly, Worsley's son John remembers as a child receiving similar kinds of advice from someone resembling Ono when the latter visited their home, probably in the 1960's.)[381] Shima described Ono's approach as more focussed on the Spirit than the physical body, and claimed that advice about psychological problems was an integral part of Ono's style of "acupuncture." Certainly one could envision an influence on Worsley both in terms of very delicate needle techniques, and in regard to the emphasis on the Mind and Spirit as more crucial issues than the Body in most cases. Shudo confirmed that Ono had travelled to a number of European acupuncture conferences, thus corroborating Worsley's version of how they met. Ono was one of Yanagiya's earliest colleagues, working with him to develop MT since 1939. He is seen in Figure 209 with Honma and Schmidt, thus further confirming the hypothesized lineage of MT teachers whose work influenced Worsley. I have tried to communicate with Ono in Japan, but he is 89 years old now, and in such poor health that his family says he cannot provide any useful information. He does leave behind him, however, an association, Tohokai, which he founded, and several publications in Japanese which may ultimately reveal more about this obscure teacher who seems to have had such a significant impact on Worsley and LA.

I've made a summary chart which includes all of the lineages I've described (Fig.210). As one can see, it's almost impossibly complex, which gives the proper feeling for how much cross-influence there has been among the different traditions. I've also drawn a simplified chart to indicate the major influences on the development of LA (Fig.211). I trust that this reconstruction meets the requirements of those who have called for an identification of the traditional sources of the LA syllabus. For a systematic presentation of the sources for the material taught in LA which I've identified in this text, see the Appendix. The main point I hope to make with this reconstruction and these flow charts is how much interaction there has been between all the teachers of the different styles of twentieth century acupuncture.

One area that I haven't discussed, and which I'd like to touch on as a post-script, is the personal charisma of the teacher or healer. Ted Kaptchuk mentioned to me, after watching Worsley at work, that he thought Worsley was the greatest shamanistic healer he had ever seen.[382] I think this is an aspect of our profession that needs to be brought out into the open, and Worsley has constantly stressed that developing the deepest possible rapport with patients, and then allowing yourself to become an instrument for forces beyond your own personal power, is what we should all be striving for. That's a good definition, as far as I'm concerned, of a shaman. The reader may remember that the shaman or wu was originally the bottom part of the character for doctor or healer, yi, the upper part containing a quivvered (non-aggressive) arrow and a right hand moving like a bird's wing which image the acupuncture practitioner.[383] (It is interesting to note both Worsley's nickname, "the Feather," and the image of Bian Que as a bird) (Fig.212). It is easy to see the shamanistic roots in Worsley's inclusion of Possession, i.e., the Seven Dragons for Seven Devils protocol, in LA. I was struck in this regard even more by his description of a Husband-Wife imbalance in a patient on whom he was consulting in the treatment for multiple sclerosis.[384] He described how hard the struggle to set things right seemed to be, and noted that the key to its ultimate resolution might have

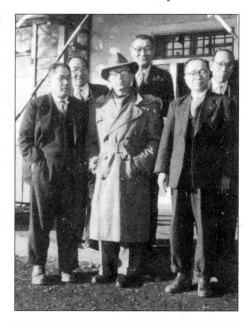

Figure 209:
ONO'S LINKAGE TO SCHMIDT
is confirmed by this photograph showing (left to right) an unidentified individual, Suzuki, Schmidt, Kimura, Honma and Ono, taken in 1953.

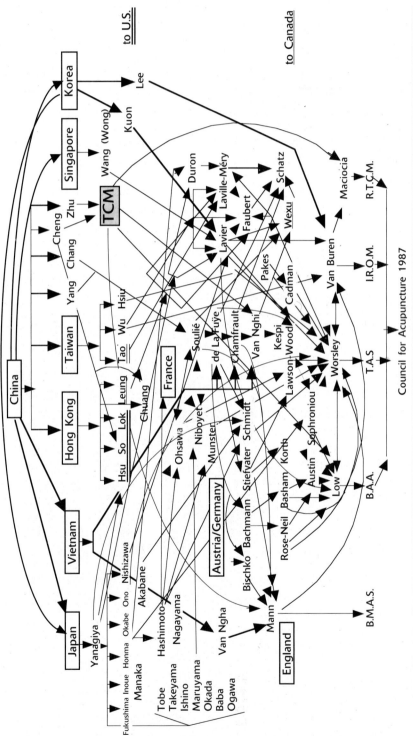

Figure 210: ACUPUNCTURE LINEAGES.

This chart, while summarizing information in the text, is a tentative reconstruction, and is not meant as a definitive version. At the very least it contains errors of omission which the author hopes the publication of this work will encourage others to begin to dispell. It has purposely been left in its original rough form in order to more accurately reflect the spirit of the author's process in tracing these lineages.

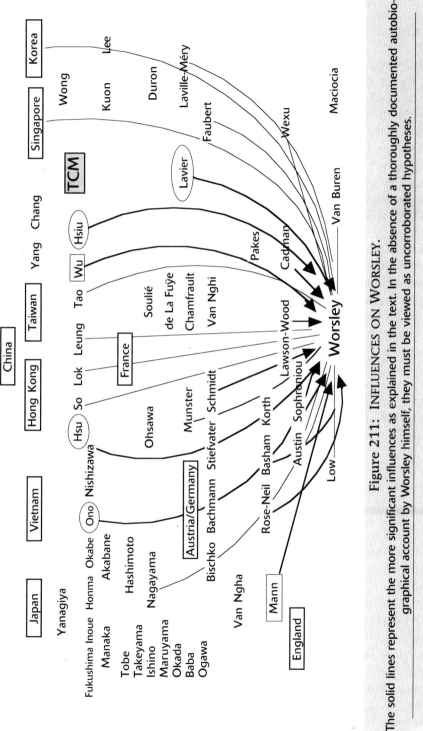

Figure 211: INFLUENCES ON WORSLEY.

The solid lines represent the more significant influences as explained in the text. In the absence of a thoroughly documented autobiographical account by Worsley himself, they must be viewed as uncorroborated hypotheses.

been the patient's prior treatment by more symptomatic approaches (by none other than Wu Wei-p'ing, and rather successfully at that, although unfortunately only lasting a matter of months) which might tragically have alerted the "wife" to impending attempts to reverse her usurpation, and allowed her to become even more firmly entrenched. This personification of all aspects of the struggle between the forces of health and those of illness, seen also in the doctrine of the Officials, is a shamanistic approach, which LA integrates successfully with the more "scientific" approaches such as the doctrine of the Five Elements which is based on the notion of systematic correspondence and resonance (gan ying), a distinction emphasized by Unschuld. I like to think that the underlying theme behind these two viewpoints is the idea of macro-cosm and microcosm reflecting each other, or as it is spelled out in TOM, the doctrine of Heaven, Earth and Man—the Three Powers. These concepts are common to both shamanism and systematic correspon-dence, and flow almost immediately from the concept of the Dao itself, however they incorporate a certain "religious" orientation, which I would like to emphasize. I would be remiss if I didn't also mention that Worsley has very strong religious convictions which have undoubtedly influenced the style of acupuncture he teaches. I won't dwell on this subject, but I believe it relates to the question of what role the healer sees himself as playing.

Worsley is known to have had a particular interest in the eso-teric Christian teachings, including those of the Essene sect.[385] In this context I should mention W.R. Morse (Fig.213), a Protestant mission-ary in China (Chengdu, Sichuan) who wrote at least three books touch-ing on Chinese medicine in the period from 1928 to 1934. He is of interest because in addition to focussing on the moral force of Christianity in healing, he specifically mentions the terms "body, mind and spirit," "causative factor of disease," and the "Officials," all of which are "technical terms" used in LA. The latter term Morse attribut-es to Zhang Yuan-su[386] (c. 1186) whom he claims used it in the the-ory of the four components of herbal prescriptions: Emperor (base), Prime Minister (adjuvant), Chancellor (corrective) and Ambassador (vehicle). Morse also describes Five Element theory, and it would not be surprising if Worsley had seen one or more of his books. My first expo-sure to Morse's work was in fact in Oxford, where his *Three Crosses in the Purple Mists* was waiting to be discovered on a friend's bookshelf.

Another book from roughly the same era, Edward Hume's *The Chinese Way in Medicine*, provides an additional hypothetical basis for the origin of the three special circumstances in LA that take precedence over Five Element treatment: Husband-Wife imbalances, Demonic Possession and Aggressive Energy. In one paragraph, Hume presents a schema that might be describing these very situations:[387]

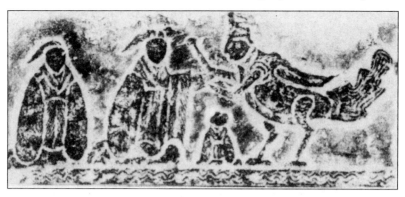

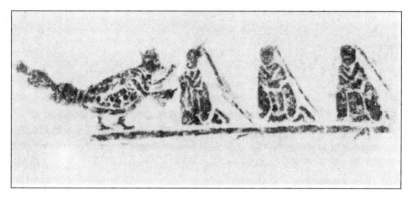

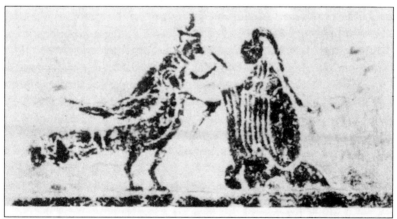

Figure 212: THE BIRD-MAN OF SHANDONG.
These Han dynasty stone reliefs have been interpreted as depicting Bian Que, whose legendary career was described in Chapter Four. They show him taking patients' pulses and performing acupuncture in the guise of a human-headed bird. The power to transform oneself into an animal is frequently encountered in shamanistic traditions.

"The physician now has all the diagnostic material in hand, and proceeds to ask himself three questions: (1) Is this illness due to a loss of balance between the Yin and the Yang, those primal forces that represent the opposing elements in the universe? (2) Are there evil spirits present whose hostility has resulted in disease? (3) Are there organic disturbances due to heat or cold, to dry conditions or damp, or to other influences in the environment that are known to be capable of producing disease?"

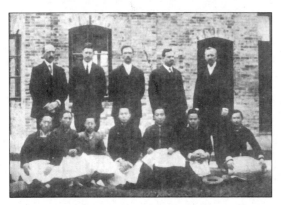

Figure 213: W.R. MORSE
(standing, fourth from the left) a Protestant missionary in China whose publications on Chinese medicine reflected a sensibility and terminology that appeared later in LA.

While this quotation is hardly more than suggestive, it would certainly be of interest to know more about Worsley's reading habits, both religious and secular.

Before leaving the subject of religion, I want to mention Dr. Edward Bach[388] (Fig.214) (1886–1936) who developed the system of flower remedies that bear his name, and which were included in my coursework at Leamington. Bach, who like Worsley grew up in Warwickshire, reached

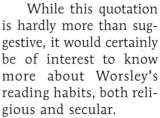

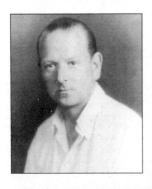

his professional acme just as Worsley was entering his teens, and conceivably they could have met. Also like Worsley, Bach was a deeply religious Christian, though in a very personal way, and many of his insights reappear in Worsley's teachings. Bach emphasized the role of emotion in health above all other factors, and totally disregarded the nature of the presenting symptoms in choosing a remedy. He believed that "healing knowledge was to be

Figure 214: EDWARD BACH (1886–1936),
English physician who developed a therapeutic system of remedies derived from flowers, whose application was based solely on the patient's emotional tendencies, and not at all on the patient's named illness, nor even on its symptoms! In this asymptomatic approach it most closely resembles both LA and the cited teachings of Ohsawa.

gained, not through man's intellect, but through his ability to see and accept the natural simple truths of life."[389] By intensive self-development, he became able to see and to hear things of which he had not been conscious hitherto. He considered himself only as the instrument through which remedies came.

In regard to the shamanistic approach to practice, I'd like to end my tale with two anecdotes, one about Bach and the other about Worsley. One evening, Bach was called to see a child who had a painful wart on one of her fingers, and this kept her awake and crying for several nights; nothing seemed to ease her. Bach took her on his knee and held the little hand, then said: "Now put her to bed, she'll sleep tonight. Her finger is healed." Her mother put her to bed, and on looking at the finger found the wart had disappeared![390] One of Worsley's first American students related a story of how Worsley had treated a little boy at Esalen who had cancer. It was the most intense and moving treatment she had ever seen him do, lasting quite a long time, but involved no needles—simply touching the child.[391] Although there was no follow-up available, the incident itself gives clear evidence of Worsley's shamanistic bent. It would be hard to imagine that he was not influenced in this regard by Bach as a role model.

I began this story with the work of George Ohsawa who was also a tremendously charismatic figure whom I believe could have equally well been described as a shamanistic healer. He had numerous miraculous cures attributed to him, and he's left behind a dedicated group of followers of his path—macrobiotics. I think you can catch a glimpse of his charismatic potential in this picture of him (Fig.215) in Paris in 1920. I'm including it, not only because I find it to be a stirring picture, but also to sound a cautionary note, because taking on the shamanistic role, accepting rapport and trust at the deepest level, can be as destructive if it is abused as it can be healing if used properly. To illustrate this, I'd like to use Ohsawa himself as an example. In the years before World War II, he adopted rabid anti-semitic views, and even applauded Hitler's treat-

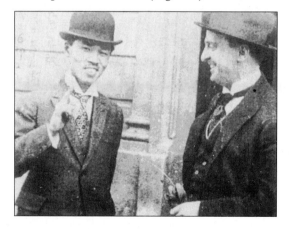

Figure 215: GEORGE OHSAWA IN PARIS in 1920. At the time he was still known as Sakurazawa Nyoitchi, and did not westernize his name until 1947.

ment of the Jews[392] and he was not alone in this—being joined in these right-wing extremist views by his friend Nakayama, whose book Ohsawa and Soulié de Morant translated into French.[393] They influenced many people in Japan, if not in the West, with these perverted ideas. On a more personal level, Ohsawa's extremist views about nutrition actually resulted in the death of one of his own children.[394] My point is that accessing shamanic powers is ethically neutral. Being an acupuncturist or a proponent of traditional Oriental medicine doesn't make one automatically good. It's what we choose to do with our special gifts that determines their ultimate effect. In closing, I'd like to bring back into the reader's minds the visions of Yanagiya (Fig.216) and his student Tobe (Fig.217) who both spent their lifetimes working to foster a spirit of open-mindedness, honest research, sharing unstintingly of themselves, along with respect and even reverence for classical tradition. I'm sure that if we all keep this vision in our mind, the acupuncture which we create in the future will be an honor to its great tradition, and a boon to all mankind.

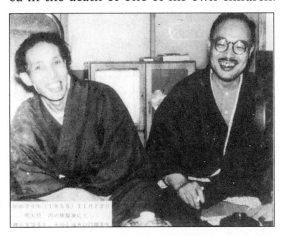

Figure 216: YANAGIYA SOREI
(right) and his disciple Maruyama in 1955, four
years before his demise.

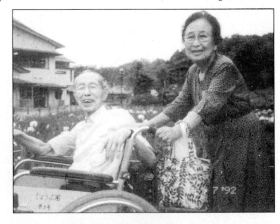

Figure 217: TOBE SOSHICHIRO
with his wife in 1992. His irrepressible spirit has kept him an active contributor to this research up until the moment it was ready for publication.

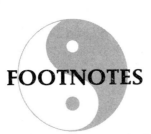

FOOTNOTES

1.   All books and articles referred to in this text can be found in the bibliography, listed alphabetically by the author's (or editor's) name.

2.   There were numerous earlier references to, and uses of acupuncture, in the West, but they were not based on a comprehension of TOM to provide an underlying coherent philosophy. They would not therefore qualify as "traditional" acupuncture, a term which I will explain in Chapter One.

3.   Flaws, et. al., p. 4; Flaws-2; Firebrace; Hicks.

4.   Moxa is an herbal substance made from the dried leaves of the wormwood plant, Artemesia vulgaris. It is often burned in small amounts at the location of acupuncture Points to stimulate them in a slightly different way than by using needles. This therapeutic burning of moxa is called moxibustion and the common Chinese term for acupuncture, "zhen jiu," actually means "acupuncture - moxibustion," reflecting how intimately these two modes of therapy are interconnected.

5.   The most reader-friendly introduction to acupuncture, which happens to have an LA slant, is the book by Peter Mole (see bibliography). The more ambitious reader should next tackle Ted Kaptchuk's *"Web,"* which is the most readable introduction to TCM. Finally, an old "classic" that predates the schism between LA and TCM, and which is still an excellent primer on acupuncture is the first book by Felix Mann, which may necessitate a trip to the library.

6.   The model based on the Circle is an elaboration of ideas first proposed by Liu Yan-chi in the *Essential Book of Traditional Chinese Medicine* which I helped to edit.

7.   Depending on the context and orientation of the author, different sources refer to one (Qi), two (Qi and Blood), three (Qi, Blood and Fluid), four (Qi, Blood, Fluid and Essence) or five (Qi, Blood, Fluid, Essence and Spirit) fundamental substances. Examples of each of these usages can be found sequentially in Bischko, p. 13; Lee and Bae, p. 28; *Essentials,* pps. 36-38; Chu and Chu, p. 14; O'Connor and Bensky, pps. 8-10.

8.   For an early review, see Eckman-1. A more up to date account can be found in the first chapter of Stux and Pomeranz's book *Acupuncture Textbook and Atlas* written by the second of the two authors.

9.   See, for example, the proceedings of the *National Symposium of Acupuncture and Moxibustion and Acupuncture Anesthesia* in Beijing in 1979, which alone cited well over 100,000 cases of various ailments treated by acupuncture with highly favorable results.

10.   These ancient characters (气 and 氣) are the ones given by Faubert, p. 22. A different set of ancient characters for Yin and Yang (陰 and 陽) are given in Lavier-6, p.30, and Lavier's versions are clearly the precursors of the characters (陰 and 陽) which are used in all the medical classics. Faubert's versions interestingly, are closer to the simplified modern characters (阴 and 阳) which are used in TCM.

11.   The Solid Organs are called Zang in Chinese, while the Hollow Organs are called Fu. The Solid Organs are the Heart, Pericardium, Spleen, Lungs, Kidneys and Liver, and are Yin in nature by comparison to the more Yang Hollow Organs, which are the Small Intestine, Triple Heater, Stomach, Large Intestine, Bladder and Gall bladder.

12.   'ba gang bien zheng' in Chinese. Various authors have translated this phrase alternatively as the Eight Principal Syndromes (Xie and Huang), Eight Leading Principles (Hoizey and Hoizey), Eight Parameters (O'Connor and Bensky), Eight Principal Patterns (Kaptchuk-1) and Eight Diagnostic Categories (Kutchins).

13.   Needle techniques to foster tonification or its opposite, dispersion or sedation, have

been meticulously described in both classical and modern texts. For the moment this subject is beyond the scope of the present work, but will be mentioned again when it bears on the historical issues to be discussed.

14.   Ling Shu, Chap. 8. Lu, p. 725.

15.   Su Wen, Chap. 26. Veith, p. 222.

16.   The Five Elements is a translation of the Chinese term 'wu xing'. Many authors have objected to this translation as being inaccurate, and insist on a more process-oriented translation, such as Five Movements or Five Phases. Both connotations are actually present in the Chinese use of the term wu xing. I will stick with the Five Elements translation out of respect for its long history of prior usage, especially with the focus of this study on LA in which the term Five Elements serves practically as a trademark. The reader is encouraged however, to constantly envision the other connotations whenever the term Five Elements is used.

17.   The Akabane test is a measurement of the comparative heat sensitivity of the Points on the tips of the fingers and toes on which are located the beginnings or endings of the various Meridians. It was developed by the late Japanese acupuncturist Akabane Kobe who will be mentioned again in Chapter Five.

18.   The methodology of transferring Qi via the Five Elements will also be the subject of a more detailed discussion in Chapter Five.

19.   Hucker, p. 22.

20.   Zhuang Zi, Chapter 7. See note 21.

21.   The names Shu and Hu have been variously translated as Suddenness and Quickness (Giradot), Heedless and Sudden (Legge), Change and Uncertainty (Needham and Feng) and Act on Your Hunch and Act in a Flash (Merton). The Chaos embodied in Emperor Hun-tun has survived into modern times as the Chinese won-ton, a culinary delicacy made from multiple ingredients all mashed together "chaotically," and wrapped in a sheet of dough before being cooked. This cultural tidbit was noted by Needham, p. 120.

22.   Steiner, p. ix.

23.   The number of holes in this poem includes the traditional seven in the head (two eyes, two ears, two nostrils and one mouth) plus the two in the lower body (anus and urethra), making Han Shan's version delightfully earthy.

24.   Translation by Burton Watson as cited in Giradot, p. 21. Now available in a Shambhala edition.

25.   The dividing line between legend and history is drawn at different times by various scholars. My presentation follows that of K.C. Wu, who provided most convincing evidence and a rationale for his choice in his book cited in the bibliography.

26.   Hoe, J. p. 32.

27.   Also known as the *Dao De Jing*; there are numerous English translations, my own favorite being the 76 page simple and poetic one by Bynner.

28.   Waley, p. 83.

29.   Wu, K.C., p. 87.

30.   Echoing Yu's sentiment, Sun Si-miao, probably the most celebrated physician of the seventh century, remarked, "I consider the pain and misery of the patient to be my own." Cited in Chuang, p. 36 and Hsia et. al., p. 44 as an excerpt from *Thousand Ducat Prescriptions*.

31.   The Yi Jing is one of the Confucian Classics. The most widely acclaimed translation is that of Wilhelm and Baynes.

32.   Based on Wu, K.C. pps. 61 and 64.

33.   Scholars disagree about the date of the *Nei Jing*, opinions ranging from 200 A.D. to 475 B.C., with most agreement between 100 and 300 B.C. See Kaptchuk-1, p, 358, Hsu and Peacher, p. 17; and Chuang-2, p. 21; Lu and Needham, pps. 69 and 89; *ACTS*, p. 338; Xie and Huang, p. 369.

34.   Lu and Needham, p. 73; *ACTS*, p. 345; Chuang-2, p. 6.

35. Lee and Bae, p. 3; Wang-1, p. 85.

36. The *Shan Hai Jing* is though to date from about 500 B.C., but contains material from prior to 1,000 B.C. - see Lu and Needham, p. 70; Schiffeler, p. II.

37. Su Wen, 14; The *Shuo Wen Jie Zi*, (*Explaining the Graphs and Explicating their Combinations*), an authoritative Han dynasty dictionary, says "bian" means "curing of diseases by pressing with a stone."

38. Qiu, p. 2.

39. Chuang-2, p. 5; Lu and Needham, p. 73.

40. *ACTS*, p. 345.

41. Qiu, p. 2.

42. Lavier-6, p. 22.

43. Wieger, p. 5; Wu, K.C., p. 26 and 31.

44. Hsu and Peacher, p. 7.

45. Wu, K.C., p. 31.

46. Lavier-6, p. 17.

47. Covell, J.C., p. 21.

48. Unschuld-1, p. 35 points out that during the Shang dynasty, the wu were the leaders or chiefs of their clan, and were responsible for the sacrifices to the deified ancestor, Di. This practice carried over into the Zhou dynasty before dying out. See also Porter, p. 19: "Ch'i (shaman emperor of the Xia dynasty) was the successor of another shaman, Yu the Great. When Yu founded the Xia dynasty around 2200 B.C., he ordered his officials to compile a guide to the realm. The result was the *Shan Hai Jing (Classic of Mountains and Seas)* to which later emperors added as their knowledge of the realm's mysteries increased."

49. Covell, A.C.-2, p. 70.

50. Hume, pps. 60-61.

51. Lu and Needham, p. 78; Needham, p. 134.

52. Chuang-2, p. 6.

53. Unschuld-1, p. 45.

54. Covell, J.C. p. 44.

55. Lu and Needham, p. 78.

56. Covell, J.C. p. 21.

57. Covell, A,C.-2, p. 10.

58. Wu, K.C. p. 11; Needham, p. 306-307.

59. Needham, p. 327.

60. Eckman-2.

61. Hyatt, p. 18; Wu, K.C., p. 54.

62. Hoizey and Hoizey, p. 5.

63. *Shen Nong's Pharmacopeia* was probably written around the second century B.C. - See *ACTS* p. 352.

64. A "radical" is a part of a Chinese ideogram which frequently conveys information about its meaning, as opposed to its pronunciation, which latter aspect is frequently conveyed by a "phonetic" component.

65. Wu, K.C., p. 57. Interestingly, Gongsun is the name of the acupuncture Point Sp. 4, which commands the opening of the Extraordinary Meridian Chong Mo, which is believed to be the main pathway for distribution of Ancestral or Original energy (Yuan Qi) and Essence (Jing) which we receive from our parents.

66. Hucker, p. 26. Also note the following quotation from Porter, p. 21, "When Yu the Great founded the Xia dynasty near the end of the third millenium, it could only have been on the basis of these Yang Shao-Lungshan cultures that he and his ministers compiled the Shan Hai Jing, the shaman's guide to the sacred world."

67. The Five Premier Emperors are Huang Di, Di Ku, Zhuan Xu, Yao and Shun.

68. Lao Zi was situated in the sixth century B.C. in the *Historical Records*, Chap. 63, but some scholars date him as late as the fourth century B.C. which is also the estimat-

ed date of Zhuang Zi. Porter, p. 37 notes that "among the areas in which Lao Zi possessed uncommon knowledge was the realm of ritual, a not unusual specialization for someone whose spiritual ancestors were shamans.

69. 'Jia' means house, family or school.
70. 'Jiao' means a religious sect.
71. Needham, p. 56.
72. e.g., *Guan Yin Zi*, an eighth century Taoist text cited by Needham, p. 73 says, "Those who are good at archery learnt from the bow and not from Yi the Archer. Those who manage boats learnt from boats and not from Wo (the legendary mighty boatman). Those who can think learnt for themselves, and not from the Sages."
73. Szuma Chien, pps. 71-72; De Woskin pps. 11-12.
74. Needham, pps. 280-281.
75. ibid. p. 286.
76. Levenson and Schurmann, p. 43.
77. Lu and Needham, p. 157.
78. Liu and Liu, p. 209.
79. ibid. p. 209.
80. Wong and Wu, p. 41.
81. *Su Wen*, 13. Author's adaptation based on Lu-1, p. 83. Jiudai Ji was legendarily contemporaneous with Shen Nong. As Qi Bo learned medicine by studying the treatment of patients two generations past, i.e., in the time of Shen Nong, the implication is that Jiudai Ji was the originator of TOM. This hypothesis is givien in Chuang-2, p. 22.
82. *Su Wen*, 13 abridged from Lu-1, p. 82.
83. It should be noted, however, that the traditional view is to regard the most ancient of practices as the highest, and thus spiritual healing and its companion, education in the correct way of life (Dao), are the epitome of therapeutics, although no longer sufficient.
84. Lu and Needham, p. 78, quoting the *Tso Chuan*.
85. ibid., p. 80, quoting the *Historical Record*; Chuang-2, pps. 24-25; Hsu and Peacher, pps. 13-15; also known as Qin Yue-ren. According to Liaw (p. 31), Bian Que in ancient Chinese merely meant "practitioner," and so was clearly not his original name.
86. Hume, p. 77.
87. According to Si-Ma Qian's biography of Bian Que, which is cited by both De Woskin, p. 20 and Hoizey and Hoizey, p. 32. Liaw (p. 32) specifies that the assassin was hired by the Imperial Physician, Lee-peng.
88. Zhuang Zi, Chap. 29.
89. Mencius, Chap. 4., cited in Lu and Needham, p. 175.
90. *Su Wen*, Chap. 12.
91. Kaptchuk-1, p. 358.
92. The best translation being that of Unschuld-4.
93. Lu and Needham, p. 115.
94. Matsumoto and Birch, p. 114; Hashimoto, p. 42; Lee and Bae, p. 208; Back, pps. 24-25; Bischko, p. 33; Chamfrault, pps. 150-151; Lawson-Wood-4, pps. 64-66; and Connelly, p. 114.
95. *Essentials*, p. 56-57; Chu and Chu, p. 31; O'Connor and Bensky, p. 28; and NACA, Lesson 13, pps. 2-4 which gives the clearest description of the origin and significance of these two contrasting styles of pulse diagnosis.
96. Levenson and Schurmann, p. 79.
97. Also known as Cang Gong or Master of the Granary—his office in Shandong Province.
98. Liu and Liu, p. 200; Xie and Huang, p. 343; Lu and Needham, pps. 106-110 present an account of his case histories; An interesting sidelight on the history of corporal punishment can be found in Wallnöfer and Von Rottauscher, pps. 30-31, who relate

the politically motivated sentencing of Chunyu Yi to having his limbs cut off, but Emperor Wen Ti pardoned him on account of the filial piety of Chunyu's daughter, who offered herself as a slave to the Emperor.   Wen Ti was so moved by her example that he later abolished punishment by maiming for the duration of his reign.

99. Chuang-2, pps. 25-26.
100. ibid. p. 27. Other accounts of Guo Yu can be found in Lu and Needham, p. 115 and Hoizey and Hoizey, pps. 39-40.
101. For the opposing view, see Mann-5, pps. 28 and 36-38.
102. Lu and Needham, pps. 117-118. I should mention, however, that the succinct manner of describing Hua's miraculous results is part of a Chinese cultural tradition in which poetic glorification seems to play a significant role, this comment applying equally to all those mentioned in this chapter.
103. "Jia Ji" means "Lining the Spine," as noted in O'Connor and Bensky, p. 217.
104. *Essentials*, p. 291.
105. A symbolic reversal of roles? Cao Cao did eventually die in great pain from what was most probably a brain tumor, as related in Duke, p. 35.
106. Chuang-2, p. 29. For a contrary opinion, see Flaws' editor's preface in Yang-1. Hua did, however, have two disciples who may have maintained his lineage of practices. Wu Pu was noted for his mastery of therapeutic exercizes, while Fan A specialized in acupuncture, and was reputed to have used very deep needling techniques, sometimes exceeding five inches, with excellent results. See Liaw (p. 33), Hoizey and Hoizey (p. 47) and Chuang (p. 29).
107. Cheng et. a., p. 14.
108. Chan, W.T. p. 305; partially translated by Wallacker.
109. Levenson and Schurmann, pps. 122-124; Liu, D.-1, pps. 221-23.
110. De Woskin, 1993 as interpreted by Flaws in the editor's preface to Yang-1, p. xi.
111. Levenson and Schurmann, p. 127.
112. Liu, D.-1, p. 21.
113. Needham, p. 330; Maspero, pps. 536-537.
114. Hoizey and Hoizey, pps. 41-42; Bensky et. al. pps. 3-4; Unschuld-1, p. 41; Hsu and Peacher, pps. 10-11.
115. *ACTS*, p. 352 cites the *Shi Jing* (*Book of Odes*) and *Shan Hai Jing* in this regard, the latter naming 120 drugs of vegetable, animal and mineral origin and describing their effects in treating and preventing diseases.
116. Lu-2, pps. 18-19.
117. Kaptchuk-1, p. 359; Hsu and Peacher, p. 41; Na, p. 2 claimed that this work was based on the lost four volume *Commentary of Lei Kung*, a contemporary of Qi Bo and Yu Fu.
118. Kaltenmark, p. 126.
119. Hsu and Peacher, p. 37.
120. Kaltenmark, p. 131.
121. Wong and Wu, p. 70. They note that during the Tang dynasty, approximately one third of the Chinese rulers died from alchemical experiments!
122. Zhang was himself a practicing Daoist as noted by Liu D.-1, p. 119.
123. See Zhang in the bibliography for English versions of these two works.
124. Chuang-2, p. 30.
125. *ACTS*, p. 342; Xie and Huang, p. 343.
126. Zhang-2, p. 3.
127. Lu-2, p. 37.
128. Zhang-1, p.3.
129. ibid, p. 71 from the commentary by Otsuka Keisetsu.
130. ibid, p. 89 from the commentary by Otsuka Keisetsu; Unschuld-3, pps. 108-110; Huang-fu, pps. xxiii - xxv.
131. Zhang-1, p. 89. Otsuka cites a text called *Shang Han Lun Yi Chien Pien* of unknown authorship which traced the origin of the *Shang Han Lun* to the *Yi Jing*.
132. Eckman-2.

133. Hsu and Peacher, p. 31.
134. Lu and Needham, pps. 100 and 119.
135. Matsumoto and Birch, p. 154.
136. Hsu and Peacher, p. 33.
137. ibid. p. 33; Chuang-2, pps. 30-31; Huang-fu, p. ix.
138. Lu and Needham, p. 119; Xie and Huang, p. 344.
139. Hsu and Peacher, p. 49.
140. Wong and Wu, p. 41. They cite the dictum in *Huai-Nan Zi* that doctors cannot cure their own complaints.
141. Lu and Needham, p. 129.
142. Liu and Liu, p. 201.
143. *Prescriptions Left by the Ghost of Liu Juan-zi* by Gong Qing-xuan, cited in Kaptchuk-1, p. 359.
144. Literally, *Discussions on the Origins of Symptoms in Illness* as cited in Kaptchuk-1, p. 359, this work is more commonly referred to by its patronymic title—see Chuang-2, p. 35.
145. Lu and Needham, p. 121.
146. ibid. p. 122.
147. ibid. p. 131; Hsu and Peacher, pp. 56-59. Two models were cast, one of which was lost in the Southern Sung dynasty and the other being in the National Museum in Tokyo where it can be seen only by special arrangement. Fig.78A is from a private viewing attended by the author.
148. Lu and Needham, p. 127.
149. Wang Tao was not however a physician, but had learned medicine from books, friends and practically in the course of nursing his sick mother. See Wong and Wu, p. 84.
150. ibid. p. 177; Chuang-2, p. 40.
151. Hsu and Peacher, p. 55.
152. Duke, pps. 32-33.
153. Ozaki, p. 37; Kaptchuk-1, p. 358.
154. Porkert, p. 56.
155. The Five Phases are primarily correlated with the Organs or Officials, while the Six Energies (Wind, Cold, Damp, Dry, Heat and Fire) are primarily correlated with the Meridians (the Six Levels of Yin and Yang), so phase energetics helped to develop a rationale for both the climatic etiology of illnesses and their treatment via acupuncture.
156. Porkert, pps. 56-59; Lu and Needham, pps. 139-140.
157. Kaptchuk-1, p. 361; Unschuld-1, pp. 175-177.
158. Also known as Liu Shou-zhen.
159. Unschuld-1, pps. 172-173; Liu and Liu, p. 202; Hsu and Peacher, p. 67; Hoizey and Hoizey, pps. 93-94.
160. Personal communication from Paul Lepron, M.D., 1992, a colleague and disciple of the late French acupuncturist Jacques Lavier. See also Kaptchuk-1, p. 362.
161. And also called Li Ming-zhi.
162. Yuan Qi, also known as Source Qi.
163. Unschuld-1, pp.s 177-179; Xie and Huang, p. 350; Kaptchuk-1, p. 362; Hsu and Peacher, pps. 71-73; Chuang-2, p. 45.
164. Hoizey and Hoizey, p. 95.
165. Also known as Zhang Zi-he.
166. Unschuld-1, pps. 174-175; Xie and Huang, p. 350; Hsu and Peacher, p. 69; Hoizey and Hoizey, pps. 96-97; Dale and Cheng, p. 95.
167. And also called Chu Yen-hsiu and Zhu Zhen-xiang.
168. "Princely" Fire (jun huo) relates mostly to the functions of the Heart and Small Intestine, while "Ministerial" Fire (xiang huo) relates mostly to the functioning of the Pericardium and Three Heater, although this term is also used to refer to "Fire"

aspects of the functioning of any other Organs, e.g., Liver, Kidney and Gall bladder.

169. Unschuld-1, p. 198; Xie and Huang, p. 353; Kaptchuk-1, p. 362; Chuang-2, pp.s 49-50; Hsu and Peacher, pps. 75-77; Hoizey and Hoizey, pps. 97-98.

170. Hoizey and Hoizey, p. 94; Unschuld-3, pp. 102-104. Zhang Yuan-su was also known as Zhang Jie-gu (Xie and Huang, p. 349), and he was Li Gao's principal teacher (Chuang, p. 45). He is credited with introducing the use of the twelve Jing-Well Points for the treatment of stroke, an advance that exemplifies his teaching that doctors must treat Oriental medicine as an evolving discipline, and that new disorders required new methods of treatment. He had a strong influence on the Four Great Schools, not only teaching Li Gao, but also personally curing Liu Wan-su of a stubborn case of typhoid fever. Another of his disciples, Wang Hao-gu (1200-1264) emphasized the fundamental role of the source or Yuan Points in acupuncture therapy, and the use of CV4 and CV6 to tonify spleen Yang (Dale and Cheng, pps. 96-97).

171. Kaptchuk-2, pps. xxxi and xxxv.

172. Cheng et. al., p. 116.

173. Lu and Needham, pps. 141, 148-149.

174. Also known as Dou Jie. He was a high ranking Official at the Imperial Court, as well as both a noted surgeon and acupuncturist (Liaw, p. 54). See also Dale and Cheng, pp. 96-97.

175. Lu and Needham, p. 137; Hoizey and Hoizey, p. 98; Chuang-2, pps. 546-547.

176. Jiang Yi-jun.

177. Ma Kan Wen, p. 98.

178. Lu and Needham, pps. 156-157.

179. Also known as Gao Mei-gu.

180. Chuang-2, pp. 56-57.

181. Matsumoto and Birch, p. 159; Chuang-2, p. 56.

182. Ma Ken-Wen, p. 98. Earlier Ming dynasty authors, such as Chen Hui (c. 14th to 15th c.) had proposed protocols for the needle techniques of tonification and sedation that used reversed laterality in treating males and females (Dale and Cheng, p. 99).

183. Xie and Huang, p. 355; Dale and Cheng, p. 102. *Yi Xue Ru Men* was translated into French by Soulié de Morant as *Le Diagnostic par les Pouls radiaux*, and published posthomously in 1983.

184. Also known as Zhang Jing-yue, Chang Hui-ching, Dong Yi-zi and Zhang Di-huang.

185. Liu, Y. p. 231.

186. Chuang-2, p. 60-61; Unschuld-1, pps. 199-200, 220-221; Bensky et. al., p. 11; Kaptchuk-1, p. 176; Hoizey and Hoizey, p. 114.

187. Lu and Needham, p. 159; Chuang-2, p. 57; Hoizey and Hoizey, p. 116; Xie and Huang, pps. 356-357; Dale and Cheng, p. 103.

188. Also known as Zhao Shu-xuan and Zhao Yi-ji.

189. Unschuld-1, pps. 211-212; Xie and Huang, p. 364; Hoizey and Hoizey, pps. 146-147.

190. Also known as Li Bin-hu and Li Dong-bi.

191. Hsu and Peacher, pps. 79-81; Kaptchuk-1, p. 363; Xie and Huang, p. 356; Chuang-2, pps. 54-55; Hoizey and Hoizey, pps. 120-127.

192. *Qi Jing Ba Mai Gao* and *Bin Hu Mai Xue*.

193. Also known as Wang Sheng-zhi and Wang Shi-shan. See Xie and Huang, p. 354; Hoizey and Hoizey, pps. 115, 117; Dale and Cheng, p. 101.

194. Lu and Needham, pps. 149, 158; Chuang-2, pps. 55-56.

195. Also known as Zhao Yang-gui.

196. Xie and Huang, p. 358; Unschuld-1, pps. 200-202; Hoizey and Hoizey, pps. 113-114; Kaptchuk-1, p. 364.

197. Hoizey and Hoizey, pps. 114 and 115.

198. Also known as Li Shi-cai.

199. Unschuld-1, pps. 202-203; Xie and Huang, p. 360.

200. Also known as Wu You-ke. See Xie and Huang, p. 359; Hsu and Peacher, pps. 84-87; Hoizey and Hoizey, pps. 118 - 119; Unschuld-1, pps. 205-206; Wong and Wu, p. 128.

201. Lu and Needham on p. 270 cite the work of the Dane Jacob de Bondt in that year as deserving priority.

202. Hoizey and Hoizey, p. 119.

203. The Four Divisions are Wei, Qi, Ying and Xue, or Defense Level, Energy Level, Nutritional Level and Blood Level. This theory parallels for heat diseases the Six Stages theory of the Shang Han Lun developed for cold diseases.

204. Also known as Ye Gui and Xiang-yan. See Xie and Huang, p. 361; Hoizey and Hoizey, p. 138; Hsu and Peacher, pps. 90-93. A charming anecdotal account of his career is given in Wong and Wu, pps. 149-150, including his final advice to his sons, "To be a practitioner one must be born with brains, read extensively, otherwise one will surely kill people." I find this statement to be a healthy counterpoint to the oft-stated claim that acupuncture and Chinese medicine have no side effects, and are thus inherently superior to Western medicine with its iatrogenic (doctor-caused) diseases.

205. Also known as Wu Tang. See Xie and Huang, p. 365; Kaptchuk-1, p. 365; Hoizey and Hoizey, p. 140.

206. Flaws-1, p. 281.

207. Liu, Y., p. 231.

208. Sivin, p. 330.

209. ibid. p. 112.

210. ibid. p. 175.

211. Lu and Needham, p. 160.

212. Lok Yee-kung, personal communication, 1992.

213. Lu and Needham, p. 160.

214. Hoizey and Hoizey, p. 133.

215. Lu and Needham, p. 160; Ma, p. 98.

216. AOCA, p. 6; Chang-2, p. 16.

217. Crozier, p. 36.

218. Unschuld-1, p. 250.

219. AOCA, pps. 6-7; Wong and Wu, p. 161. The 1929 prohibition of Chinese medicine was vigorously opposed by its practitioners, who met on March 17 of that year to plan a protest. They formally appealed to Chairman Chiang Kai-Shek who reversed the prohibition. Since then, March 17 has been celebrated as Chinese medicine day, as related in Liaw, p. 73.

220. Unschuld-1, p. 251.

221. AOCA, p. 7.

222. Unschuld-1, p. 251; Mao's personal role in the resurrection of traditional medicine is a subject shrouded in rumor, exacerbated by the secrecy maintained by all members of his inner circle. In my research I have uncovered two reports from respected figures in the acupuncture world (Dr. Maurice Mussat in France and Shen-ping Liang, Vice-President of the American Association of Acupuncture and Oriental Medicine) claiming that Mao was successfully treated with acupuncture for a serious medical problem (Parkinson's disease was one speculation) just at the time when TCM was first emerging as an official government supported system of health care, and that Mao's experience was a crucial factor in this development. Neither source, however, was able to offer any corroboration, both being based on lost newspaper and magazine articles, as related to me in personal communications. Contemporary historians in China are unaware of this episode, and doubt its authenticity—personal communciations from both Cai Jing-feng and the late Li Zhi-sui, Mao's personal physician who emphatically denied that Mao received acupuncture treatment.

223. Mark Seem (Am J. Ac., 1986) has claimed that the English phrase, Traditional Chinese Medicine (TCM) did not even exist until the publication of the Essentials of Chinese Acupuncture (which was written in 1964, but not published until 1979 or

1980 - see Maciocia, J. Chin Med. (U.K.), 1982. Although Seem's claim is not literally true (the phrase occurring at least in these prior publications: *Basic Acupuncture Techniques* (1973), *A Barefoot Doctor's Manual* (1974) and *An Outline of Chinese Acupuncture* (1975) the latter being compiled by the Academy of Traditional Chinese Medicine!), I still concur with his major point, that among Western practitioners of acupuncture, "TCM" did not become a familiar label until after *Essentials of Chinese Acupuncture* was published. Earlier English language books on acupuncture, such as those by Lawson-Wood and Felix Mann in the 1950's and 1960's used the phrase Chinese medicine to translate zhong yi, and only after the Chinese began publishing their own English texts did the word traditional become incorporated in this phrase.

224. Unschuld-2, p. 17.
225. Sivin, pps. 3-4.
226. Leon Hammer has published the following anecdote in *Dragon Rises, Red Bird Flies* (p. xxiv):
    On my way to Beijing airport at the end of a three-months stay, a Chinese doctor explained to me that in the early nineteen-sixties, responding to a drive by the World Health Organization to encourage the use and spread of indigenous health systems, the Chinese government brought together a group of acceptable Chinese physicians and ordered them to create "Traditional Chinese medicine" so that, under the auspices of that organization, it could be taught to the Chinese people and to foreigners. Thus ended the practice of "following a master for many years in relative servitude, and the thousands of blossoms on the tree of this medicine fell away until one was left. Anyone in the West who believes they have the 'real' Chinese medicine is living in a dangerous world of fantasy."
    The Chinese themselves have stated that "acupuncture was set up as a major course as early as the 1950's when the higher education of TCM was established."– Fu. The recently published work by Dale and Cheng provides some interesting information on contributions of twentieth century acupuncturists in China, pps. 107-115.
227. Wang-2, p. 329; Huard and Wong-2, pps. 217-219; Jarricot, H. and Wong, M. in Niboyet-4, pps. 136, 141 (in French). Some of the following material on Zhu Lian is from Liaw.
228. Flaws-1, p. 60.
229. Kaptchuk, in JCM, 17 (Jan. 1985) p. 26 stated, "The treatments that are now being used in China I think come from the 1930's, with a modification in the last ten years from that guy Chang Tan An who was the innovator of modern acupuncture in China." Liaw, p. 74, notes that Cheng had established an Institute of Acupuncture in Jiangsu as early as 1933. It was only after this first Institute was destroyed in a Japanese bombing raid, that he established a second Institute in Chengdu.
230. Huard and Wang-2, p. 217; Liaw, personal communication. One of the books Cheng translated was the twelve year clinical record of cases treated by Sawada Ken, whose work I will describe in the next chapter, as recorded by his student Bunshi Shirota.
231. According to Liaw, p. 74, after the establishment of the People's Republic, most of Cheng's students went to Hong Kong. Two of them will be discussed again in Chapter Five. The first is Chuang Yu-min, whom Liaw claims to have been a direct disciple of Cheng (p. 84). The second is Dr. James Tin-Yao So, founder of the New England School of Acupuncture, whose own teacher, Zhang Tian-qi was a direct student of Dr. Cheng. Dr. So published several books that are cited in the bibliography, and was one of the teachers Worsley visited in Hong Kong according to a personal communication from Bob Duggan, but this material awaits development in Chapter Five.
232. Palos, pps. 80, 103, 111-15, 122.
233. Huard and Wong-2, pps. 150, 219. Liaw.
234. Kaptchuk-2, pps. xxxiii-xxxiv.
235. ibid. p. xxxv.
236. Flaws et al. pps. 129, 134-135. This prescription translates as "All-inclusive Great

Tonifying Decoction."

237. Peng, p. 43.

238. Tany, p. 203; Small, p. 147.

239. Unschuld-1, p. 261.

240. Sivin, p. 145; Crozier, p. 45.

241. Shudo, p. 4.

242. Chuang-2, pps. 67-69; Hsu and Peacher, pps. 118-121.

243. Some of the methodologies which were not incorporated into LA per se were nevertheless preserved in Worsley's out of print *Acupuncturists Therapeutic Pocket Book*, affectionately known as the "little black book'.

244. Worsley has written two volumes of a text called *Traditional Acupuncture*, but these cover only the areas of Meridian and Point location and of traditional diagnosis, and in no way purport to be a comprehensive text on LA.

245. Also reported as being spelled Hsiue, Hsiu, Hsui, Shiu and Shsiu at different times, and as being pronounced "Shoo" or "Su."

246. With Bob Duggan, c. 1973 and with Charles Fox, 1978. Both related to me in person. Also a similar account appears in Trad. Acup. Soc. J. 1, March, 1987, p. 1, by Worsley's son John.

247. The Acupuncture Association Newletter (U.K.) of October, 1966, contains a letter from Wu Wei-P'ing conferring on Worsley and Stemp the authority to examine candidates for the intermediate level of proficiency in acupuncture under Wu's seal. The examination for doctorate level was not delegated at that time, and Wu signed the letter as "your Patron and Master." The photographs, in addition to recording the ritual "bow" to both Wu and his parents, also document the presence of many of the prominent teachers of Chinese medicine at this ceremony, including Eric (Hsi-yu) Tao and Tsui Chieh, both of whom will be discussed in this chapter. In addition, other attendees whom Worsley met included Lee Huan-hsin (Director of the Chinese Medicine Research Institute), Wang Chen-xian (President of the Acupuncture Association of Taipei), Chang Kwai-fu (President of the Acupuncture Association of Taichung), Tsao Cheng-chang, Lin Xue-nu, Wu Hai-feng, Li Shu-yu, Chen Kuo-chen, Dai Yun-jiang, Tu Chuan-fu and Hsi, Y.F. A final participant will be introduced at the end of this chapter. I am indebted to Eric Tao and Luying Liaw for identifying the individuals shown, and to the College of Traditional Acupuncture (U.K.) for making these photographs available.

248. The translations from French are my own.

249. p. 42.

250. p. 37.

251. p. 38.

252. p. 45.

253. p. 50.

254. p. 51.

255. p. 47.

256. p. 71.

257. p. 60.

258. p. 72.

259. p. 73

260. p. 74.

261. p. 74.

262. pps. 74-75.

263. p. 92.

264. *L'Acupuncture et la Médecine d'Extrême Orient*, cited in the bibliography under Ohsawa.

265. My account of macrobiotics and the life of George Ohsawa is based mainly on the writings of Kotzsch.

266. Gaier, pps. 235-238.

267. Fujikawa, pps. 55-56.
268. Goethe, *Faust*, Modern Library, New York, p. 66 as cited in Kotzsch-2, p. 263.
269. Ohsawa-2.
270. Ido No Nippon, May, 1958.
271. The biographical details on Soulié de Morant are largely drawn from the articles by Choain, Jacquemin and Tim, all of which are in French, and from his own publications cited in the bibliography.
272. Artaud, pps. 127-151; 224-227.
273. Per the schema of the *Mai Jing* via the *Yi Xue Ru Men*.
274. Soulié de Morant-1, p. 66.
275. Yang, *ZJDC* III p. 324.
276. Yang, *ZJDC* IX.
277. Li, *YXRM* p. 43; Yang, *ZJDC* II p. 20.
278. Master of Heart in Yang, *ZJDC* VIII, and Envelope of Heart or Ming Men as the exit of sexual energy in gametes in Li, *YXRM* I p. 17.
279. And on passages from Yang, *ZJDC* XII.
280. In the bibliography of *L'Acuponcture Chinoise* on p.95, Soulie de Morant lists separately two works which were really the same: Tchenn tsiou ta tsiuann by Iang Tsi-che and Tchenn tsiou ta Tchreng by Iang Ko-sien.
281. This account is derived in large part from articles and letters in Ido No Nippon, an important Japanese acupuncture journal published by Mr. Tobe Soshichiro, who provided excerpts from back issues dating to the 1950's. Translation into English was generously provided by Ms. Chieko Maekawa, who helped unravel this tale. Additional details on Mme. Hashimoto were provided by her grand-daughter, Hashimoto Mariko, currently the third generation of her family practicing acupuncture at the same location in Tokyo.
282. Biographical details on Yanagiya were again supplied by Mr. Tobe, with additional material provided by Mrs. Masako Yanagiya, his second wife. Translations from Japanese were done by Chieko Maekawa.
283. Fujikawa, pp. 1-2; Ozaki, p. 2.
284. Reader et. al., p. 34.
285. Chieko Maekawa, personal communication, 1993.
286. Reader, p. 39.
287. ibid. p. 124.
288. Fujikawa, p. 3.
289. My account of Japanese medical history is to a great extent based on the work of Norman Ozaki, to be found in his doctoral thesis. Shinichiro Yamada and Hirohisa Oda of the Meiji College of Oriental Medicine also contributed to my understanding of this material.
290. Ozaki, pps. 50-51.
291. Ozaki, pps. 51-52.
292. Ozaki, pps. 198-204.
293. Ozaki, pps. 204-210.
294. Ozaki, pps. 218-224. The term which Todo used to describe the "healing crisis" was "meigen" (瞑 眩).
295. Ozaki, pps. 225-226.
296. Fujikawa, p. 28.
297. Ozaki, pps. 61-67.
298. Hirohisa Oda, personal communciation, 1992.
299. Shinichiro Yamada, personal communciation, 1992.
300. Miki Shima, personal communication, 1993.
301. Matsumoto and Birch, p. 197.
302. Miki Shima, personal communciation, 1993.

303. My information on Sawada is based on personal communications from Liaw Luying and Miki Shima between 1993 and 1995.
304. Shudo, p. 5.
305. Shudo, p. 6.
306. Sa Am was the pen-name of an anonymous Buddhist monk who wrote extensively on the practical application of Five Element theory in acupuncture treatment. In addition to influencing the Meridian Therapy school started by Yanagiya, his work was also incorporated into two contemporary styles of Korean acupuncture, Constitutional Acupuncture and Hand Acupuncture developed by Drs. Kuon Dowon and Yoo Tae-Woo respectively.
307. Matsumoto and Birch, p. 198.
308. Fukushima, p. 101.
309. Honma, 1949, referring to the Zang Organs specifically.
310. Matsumoto and Birch, p. 96; Honma, 1949; Hashimoto, 1961 (English 1966).
311. Fukushima, p. 98.
312. Matsumoto and Birch, p. ix.
313. Fukushima, p. 165.
314. ibid. p. 67.
315. Shudo, p. 1.
316. Fukushima, p. 146. Akashi (証) is equivalent to the Chinese word zheng usually translatted as "pattern" as in the "Eight Principles for Discriminating Patterns." Meridian Therapy was systematized prior to TCM.
317. personal communication, Dr. J. Bischko, 1992.
318. Monnier, p. 49.
319. ibid. p. 49. The information on Prince Buu-Loc is from Liaw.
320. Tim, p. 100.
321. The account of Yanagiya's encounter with De la Fuÿe is based on material from Ido No Nippon articles donated by Tobe and translated by Maekawa.
322. Firebrace, pps. 48-49.
323. Biographical data on Dr. Schmidt are largely derived from personal correspondence with him, supported by the 1974 doctoral thesis by J. Schmidt (no relation) which was kindly translated from German by Klaus Maaser. His demise was not mentioned in any English language publication, however the Japanese acupuncture journal Ido No Nippon devoted a 1995 issue to him in tribute.
324. In fact, it was these seminars in which Schmidt taught many non-physicians which led to his "falling out" with Felix Mann, as related to me by Dr. Mann.
325. Personal communication from Joyce and Denis Lawson-Wood, 1985.
326. Flaws-2, pps. 6-7.
327. My biographical sketch of Felix Mann is mainly derived from two sources: the Preface to his 1987 *Textbook of Acupuncture* and an interview I conducted with him in 1992.
328. The following account of the emergence of acupuncture in England is based on interviews and/or correspondence with as many of the participants as I could locate, including the following: Denis and Joyce Lawson-Wood, Felix Mann, Sidney and Pat Rose-Neil, Kenneth Basham, Nicholas Sofroniou, Dick Van Buren, Malcolm Stemp, Heribert Schmidt, Royston Low, Harry Cadman, Joseph Goodman, William Wright, Eric Welton-Johnson, Keith Lamont and Jacques Lavier. A later stratum of participants who also contributed material includes John D'Ambrosio, Geoff Foulkes, Tony Evans, Roger Newman-Turner and Stuart Watts.
329. Credit for the transmission of the Five Element tradition to England must also be given to Sofroniou and through him to Lawson-Wood who transmitted the Japanese Five Element tradition of Honma, much as Ohsawa had transmitted that

of Hashimoto to France and Germany. Also Schmidt transmitted similar material from Yanagiya and the Meridian Therapists after him to all of Europe.

330. Lavier in Wu, W.P.-1, p. 11.
331. My biographical sources for Lavier include his daughter Marie-Christine, Dr. Paul Lepron, Claude Grégory, and the following written portraits: The preface by René Alquié to Lavier's *Nei Tching Sou Wen*, the preface by René Brunet to Wu Wei-p'ing's *Chinese Acupuncture*, and the preface by Louis Lécussan to Lavier's *Bio-"Enérgetique Chinoise.*
332. Charles Fox, a jounalist whom I cited earlier as one of Worsley's interviewers, was himself treated extensively by Wu, and took that opportunity to interview Wu as well. I have listened to the original tape recordings of that interview as well as discussing Fox's recollections. Cecil Chen, an official of the British College of Acupuncture, came from the same region of China (Shanghai) as Wu, and related Wu's personal history to me. Finally, Eric Tao, whom I will discuss shortly was a close colleague of Wu's in Taiwan. These three all were emphatic in their belief that Wu did not practice, nor was likely to have taught anything similar to the Five Element transfer methodology described by Lavier.
333. Personal communication from Dr. Lepron, 1992.
334. Personal communication from Dr. Van Buren, 1992.
335. A copy of the original London course syllabus belonging to one of the participants, Dr. Paul Bird, was kindly provided to me by Vivienne Brown. It describes AE on pps. 84-85 and Five Element transfers on pps. 81-83 and 85-86.
336. Flaws-2, pps. 5-7.
337. Yang and Li, pps. 143-144.
338. Lavier-3, pps. 155-164. In French. This text also describes the Five Element transfer method on pps. 137, and 185-188.
339. All of these teachings are to be found in the 1963 course syllabus and the 1966 text cited above.
340. Lavier-5, p 49.
341. Lavier-3, pps. 67-97.
342. See Kespi's excellent text, cited in the bibliography.
343. Personal communication via Dr. Joseph Helms.
344. Dr. Leung was mentioned previously as having been visited by Worsley, when Leung was chairman of the Chinese Acupuncture and Osteopathy Institute in Hong Kong. Leung was a teacher, although probably only playing a minor role, for Lavier and Worsley. He played a more prominent part in the training of Laville-Mery and Faubert, to be introduced later. Leung later moved to Vancouver, Canada, where he established the North American College of Acupuncture. Evidence of his impact on Worsley can be found in the system of Near, Middle and Distal points which appear in Worsley's out of print *Acupuncturists Therapeutic Pocket Book*, pps. B 16-19. The complete system, called Leung's method of points prescription, of which Worsley's version is a synopsis, can be found in the Clinical Manual of the North American College of Acupuncture (NACA), pps. 204-211, compiled by Dr. Leung. Leung's use of the Five Element Command Points is quite different from that taught in LA as can be seen in his article in the Am. J. Acup. cited in the bibliography, in which many uses of these points are described, but none involving energy transfers.
345. A scholar of contemporary Chinese acupuncture, Luying Liaw, who has read all of Chuang's works in Chinese, has assured me that they contain no mention of the transfer methodology.
346. Chuang's biography is derived from his two English publications just mentioned.
347. Personal communication from Luying Liaw.
348. A true Master, with whom I have had the good fortune to study during several visits to Korea.
349. Mann-1, p. 92.

350. Sources include Shudo Denmei, Sorimachi Taiichi and Tajima Sensei, all practitioners in Japan.
351. Personal communcation from Richard Yennie.
352. Personal communication from Bob Duggan.
353. Galen Fisher, who was treated by Nagayama later went on to study LA and remarked to me on their similarities.
354. In his interview with Charles Fox, Worsley was mildly critical of Nagayama's treatment style, so in the balance he's probably a less likely source for the origin of the transfer methodology.
355. Personal communication from Jayasuriya, 1993.
356. From Jayasuriya's curriculum vitae.
357. Wang and Wong can be variant spellings of the same Chinese character.
358. WICA prospectus vi (Winter 1993) p. 5. Interestingly, certain details of Worsley's teachings appear in Wong's manuals, and nowhere else that I have discovered. E.g., "The use of a point of 'tonification' is valid only when the mother organ is in excess and a point of 'sedation' is valid only when the son is deficient."-Wong-2, p. 21. "To take the pulse, the angle of the physician's fingers is most important...This is done with the fleshy tip of the fingers, and in order to do so the nails must be filed very short. This is the only possible way to take the pulse..."- ibid, p. 6.
359. Undoubtedly, the reader has asked himself by this point, why doesn't Worsley give a full public account of his past history? Although I am in the group that has urged him to do so, at the same time I recognize one possible reason for his failure to comply. As I have shown, and will develop further, Worsley has a decidedly shamanistic bent to his nature, which might preclude him from objectifying his past. The most well-known contemporary shaman is the character Don Juan Matus in the series of books by Carlos Castaneda. Don Juan's advice to Carlos was that if he had a serious desire to become a sorcerer (shaman), he had better lose his personal history, as it would only make him vulnerable. While Don Juan did relate a few biographical items to Castaneda, they amount to about the sum total of what Worsley has revealed about himself, so a similar belief system might be operative.
360. Thambirajah's biography is based on my interview with her in 1994.
361. At the time of my visit to her in England, she was not able to locate original references which unequivocally described energy transfers or Entry and Exit Points, so this assertion remains to be documented. The traditional source of the use of Entry and Exit Points was subsequently corroborated verbally by Jeffrey Yuen, although he is also still searching his texts for a documented citation. Thambirajah's version of energy transfers across the Control cycle is from Yin Organ to Yang Organ and vice-versa, thus agreeing with Wong and Lavier.
362. Interview with Cecil Chen, 1986. This assertion was corroborated by Eric Tao during a follow-up interview in 1995 in which he explained that the original mainland text, written about 40 years ago, was contraband in Taiwan, and needed an "acceptable" author in order to be published and distributed there. Conceivably, Ed Wong could have been either the author of this text, or more likely, one of its "ghost-writers" in Wong-1.
363. De la Fuÿe started the International Acupuncture Society (S.I.A.) in 1946 and the French Acupuncture Society (S.F.A.) in 1945. The latter changed its name to French Acupuncture Association (A.F.A.) in 1966. Niboyet started the Mediterranean Acupuncture Society (S.M.A.) in 1955. A parallel group formed around Lavier, the Chinese Acupuncture Medical Society (S.M.A.C.), begun in 1978.
364. Personal communication from Mark Seem based on his conversations with Oscar Wexu.
365. Personal communication from Van Buren, 1992.
366. Personal communication from Chieko Maekawa based on articles in Ido No Nippon and supplementary material from Tobe Soshichiro.
367 Personal communication from Solange Voiret.

368. The National Confederation of Medical Acupuncture Assoiactions, founded in 1969.

369. Personal communication, J.M. Kespi, 1992.

370. E.g., Lok wrote the Foreword to Van Nghi's 1971 text, *Pathogénie et Pathologie Energétiques en Médecine Chinoise*, and was laudatory in referring to Van Nghi in a letter to me, but did not acknowledge Van Nghi as his student.

371. Personal communication from Jeffrey Yuen, a third generation Daoist priest and practitioner of Chinese medicine, 1993. The *Yellow Court Classic* dates to the second or third century A.D. and is catalogued in the Dao Cang as No. 1032, chapter 17 by Schipper, p. 251.

372. Principally Chang Bin Lee, seen in Figure 186.

373. According to Ted Kaptchuk (personal communication), the first lecture on TCM style acupuncture in the U.K. was in 1979 when he taught a five day seminar with over one hundred participants including representatives from all three British acupuncture schools, which set the groundwork for the establishment of the Register of TCM. Thus, although TCM is now probably the most well-known style of traditional acupuncture, it was historically a late-comer to the English speaking members of both the profession and the public.

374. Schmidt, H. (1964) as cited in Kajdos (1974) who related the anecdote in which Akabane discovered his new methodology.

375. Biographical material on Dr. Hsu along with documentary photographs were supplied by his daughter, Margaret Ho.

376. Information on Dr. Hsiu was provided by Luying Liaw and Eric Tao in personal communications, 1994.

377. Personal communication from Frank Sun, 1994.

378. As this book was being prepared for publication, I received a brief response from J.R. Worsley to a request that he comment on the photographs herein of the individuals I've identified as some of his putative teachers. He stated that he had had contact with Heribert Schmidt, but that he did not recognize the pictures of Hsiu Yang-chai nor of Hsu Mifoo as being his Chinese "Master." He neither acknowledged nor denied meeting Hsiu Yang-chai in 1966 and did not provide further identification of the correct Master Hsiu, leaving his identity a matter for speculation, such as that given in the preceeding textual remarks and in footnote 359. The hypothesis presented there is further strengthened by Worsley's closing remark that he did not forsee having time to allocate to an in-depth biographical interview in the foreseeable future, thus cordially, but effectively closing that line of investigations.

379. Interview with Shudo Denmei, 1992.

380. Interview with Miki Shima, 1993.

381. Interview with John Worsley, 1993.

382. Interview with Ted Kaptchuk c. 1990.

383. Analysis of ideogram by Lavier-3, p. 22.

384. This description is on a clinical guidance tape recording which Worsley sent to the patient's on-going practitioner.

385. Interview with Diane Nathan, one of Worsley's first American students, 1993.

386. Morse-1, p. 87.

387. Hume, p. 121.

388. Biographical information on Edward Bach is from the book by Weeks cited in the bibliography.

389. Weeks, p. 52.

390. Weeks, p. 109.

391. Interview with Diane Nathan, 1993.

392. Kotzsch-2, p. 76.

393. Kotzsch-2, pps. 62, 63, 75.

394. Kotzsch-2. p. 99.

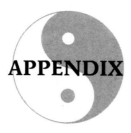

APPENDIX

**GLOSSARY OF TERMS AND CONCEPTS RELATIVELY UNIQUE TO
LA, WITH CITATIONS OF THEIR PRIOR USAGE.***

1. THE PRIMACY OF THE SPIRIT. Although all styles of traditional acupuncture make reference to Spirit or Shen (神), LA and TCM represent two opposing points of view in this regard. TCM is based on a materialist philosophy, and regards Spirit as a manifestation of organic functioning that results in the mental faculties and their outward expression (Xie and Huang, p. 39). LA is based on a more idealistic philosophy, and posits that there is something about Spirit which is transcendental, and which can never be fully stated or explained in words (*Su Wen* 26); however Spirit is considered the primary factor in giving acupuncture treatment (*Ling Shu* 8). This emphasis in the classics on the primacy of the Spirit has been most clearly maintained in the Japanese acupuncture traditions, whose early twentieth century teachers were steeped in the Shinto (Spirit Way) religious outlook (Ohsawa-1, p. 38). Worsley was exposed to this tradition both through his association with Drs. Schmidt (a student of Ohsawa and Hashimoto and many other Shinto-influenced Japanese acupuncturists) and Munster, and through his more intense association with Ono Bunkei. The equivalent Chinese tradition would be the Daoist one, which continues to guide many non-TCM trained Chinese acupuncturists around the world.

2. THE LAW OF THE FIVE ELEMENTS. Both Yin-Yang and the Five Elements or Wu Xing (五行) are referred to as theories in TCM (*Essentials of Chinese Acupuncture*, p. 11), with the former receiving much more serious consideration. The opposite emphasis is characteristic of LA which is often colloquially referred to as "Five Element acupuncture." The translation of Wu Xing as Five Elements is discussed in Footnote 16. The Five Elements were mentioned in various Chinese classics including the *Book of History* and the *Book of Rites* both of which are at least as old as the fifth century B.C., and the Five Elements are embedded in the very fabric of the *Nei Jing*, the most classical of all books about acupuncture. The *Nan Jing* which followed, was almost exclusively based on Five Element thinking. It would appear, however, that the use of the word "Law" in reference to the Five Elements is at least partially a Western development initiated by Soulié de Morant (*L'Acuponcture Chinoise* Vol. II, Chapter VIII) who translated the Chinese term fa (法) as "law," although fa can also mean "method"

* *The order of presentation follows the theory of the Circle described in Chapter One.*

which would seem to me to be the preferable choice for expressing the information Soulié de Morant translated from his Ming dynasty references (Yang, J. and Li). In any case, Worsley's use of the terms Law of Five Elements, Law of Mother-Son, Law of Husband-Wife and Law of Midday-Midnight can all be explained as derivative from Soulié de Morant's work in which specific references for each of these teachings can be found. The English terminology for these concepts is due to Felix Mann (see Mann-1), an inheritor of Soulié de Morant's lineage, whose works Worsley used in his classroom teaching.

3. THE DOCTRINE OF THE OFFICIALS. The twelve Officials are personifications of the twelve Zang Fu or Viscera and Bowels as they were originally described, with their functions and responsibilities, in *Su Wen* 8. Such personification was further developed by practitioners of the Daoist religion (Dao Jiao) who identified numerous "deities" residing within each individual, giving the Doctrine of the Officials a decidedly Daoist flavor. The English missionary William Morse used the term "Officials" to translate Zhang Yuan-su's description of the four components of an herbal prescription, and for reasons I have stated in the text, it is likely that Worsley was exposed to Morse's work. Even more certain is Worsley's exposure to Ilza Veith's translation of the *Su Wen* (Veith pps. 28-30) in which she repeatedly uses the term officials. As her partial translation of the *Su Wen* was the only English version of any of the Chinese medical classics at the time, it may have easily had a profound effect on Worsley's thinking. For further comments on personification and Daoist influences on acupuncture, see the entry on "Spirit of the Point."

4. THE SUPERFICIAL AND DEEP CIRCULATION OF ENERGY. The classics contain many descriptions of the movements of the various forms of Energy throughout the human organism. Specific pathways, the Meridians, conduct this flow of Energy through the more superficial regions of the body where it can be contacted and influenced by acupuncture needles. In addition to these Primary or Principal Meridians, there are so-called Secondary Meridians which are auxiliary pathways of two types: the first type (initially described in depth in Western texts by Chamfrault and Van Nghi although introduced in English by Mann), includes named structures such as Luo Vessels, Divergent Meridians, Tendinomuscular Meridians and Extraordinary Meridians whose flow pathways are also well described. The second type (identified as "Secondary Vessels" by Niboyet) accounts for the intangible relationships between Meridians or Organs for which there are no described structural mechanisms or pathways. Examples of this second type of Secondary Vessel include the Five Element relationships of the Creative (xiang sheng 相生) and Control (xiang ke 相克) cycles and the relationships governed by the "Laws" of Husband-Wife and Midday-Midnight. In LA, the energy flowing in the Primary Meridians is called the "Wei Circulation," while the energy circulating according to the Five Elements is called the "Deep Circulation." This division is only roughly approximate to that of The Defensive (Wei 衛) and Nourishing (Ying 營) Qi described in TCM, in which the former has an association with the Surface while the latter is more involved with the Interior. Nevertheless, it was exactly this distinction between Wei and Ying Qi that Jacques Lavier used in deciding to name the superficial circulation of Qi the "Wei Circulation" (Lavier-3, pps. 91-92), since he believed that only Wei Qi flowed in the Primary Meridians. Worsley adopted the terminology of "Wei Circulation" from Lavier under whom he had studied. It is noteworthy that TCM acupuncture focuses almost exclusively on the activities of the described Meridians on their Organs and bodily terrains, while LA focuses almost exclusively on the intangible relationships of the Five Elements, Husband-Wife, and Midday-Midnight, governed by the second type of non-localized Secondary Vessel. Citations of historical precedents for using these intangible relationships in acupuncture are given in the specific entries which follow.

   5. THE NOMENCLATURE OF THE MERIDIANS. LA uses a relatively idiosyncratic system of nomenclature of the Meridians in which the Heart, as Supreme Controller, is viewed as being analogous to the Emperor, and is labeled with the Roman numeral I to emphasize its cardinal role. The other Meridians are numbered sequentially in the traditional order acknowledged by all schools of traditional acupuncture. These other schools and all the classical texts, however, start the enumeration of the Meridians with the Lung, rather than the Heart. I have described the origin of this variant system of enumeration in Chapter Five of the text as an error made by Roger de La Fuÿe in transmitting the teachings of Soulié de Morant. In preparing the first English language book about acupuncture, Denis Lawson-Wood adopted this nomenclature from de La Fuÿe, and taught it to his English colleagues among whom were Mary Austin and J.R. Worsley. Worsley in turn propagated it, along with the justification given above, as part of LA.

   6. VARIANT POINT LOCATIONS. It should be recognized that throughout the long history of traditional acupuncture there has been no universal agreement on the exact location (nor even the exact number) of acupuncture Points. As long as Oriental medicine continues to develop according to its own dynamic (meaning without the use of "point-finders" or other instruments based on Western notions of physiology) there will be competing schools of thought about Point location. This problem is essentially no different in the twentieth century than it was in the Han dynasty. The only exception is that variations in point location due to errors in transcription and translation of texts tend to multiply over time. This mechanism may possibly be at the root of the major difference between LA and most other traditions in locating the Points on the Yin Meridians of the legs. In LA these Points tend to be located one anatomical inch higher (Worsley-2). Clearly the locations specified in LA are adopted from Chancellor's English version of Lavier's French translation of the Chinese works of Wu Wei-p'ing (Wu-1), a chain of transmission highly susceptible to such errors. All of Lavier's works in French and English, however, conform to this variant system, so if an error occurred in transmitting doctrine, it would have been by Lavier or Wu. The best explanation for this kind of systematic error would be to attribute it to a confusion regarding measurement from the internal versus the external malleolus, the former being exactly one anatomical inch higher. If the external malleolus is taken as the reference point, then LA and TCM would be in agreement. A second issue in Point location that distinguishes LA from TCM is its belief that Points can not be located merely by anatomical landmarks, but must be palpated for their exact location. This doctrine is common in the Japanese acupuncture tradition which was strongly influenced by blind practitioners, and indeed Worsley's teacher Ono was a graduate of an acupuncture school for the blind.

7. THE CAUSES OF ILLNESS. Both LA and TCM teach the theory of etiology elaborated by Chen Yen in 1174, in which disease causes are divided into exogenous, endogenous and miscellaneous categories. The differences between LA and TCM in this regard relate to their unequal emphasis in applying this theory. LA is focused around the endogenous causes of illness, which are the unbalanced emotional factors in a person's life. Although there are are traditionally "seven emotions," these endogenous causes of disease are in practice limited to five, since they are classically described as operating according to the Law of the Five Elements. The exogenous causes of illness, which are the excessive climatic factors, are only briefly mentioned, with an explanation that in modern times we struggle less with inadequate food, clothing and shelter than at any other time in the past; however this justification for LA's focus on the endogenous factors is in conflict with its claim to be the classical style of acupuncture practiced in antiquity, when presumably the relative influence of exogenous and endogenous factors was reversed. TCM on the other hand, is focused primarily around the exogenous climatic factors. These six exogenous factors are traditionally associated with the six levels of Yin and Yang, rather than with the Five Elements, which is consistent with TCM's philosophical dependence on Yin Yang as opposed to Five Element theory. Thus Wind, Cold, Damp, Heat, Dryness and Fire are all common etiological mechanisms in TCM although they are rarely mentioned in LA. This stylistic emphasis on one or another etiological category is reminiscent of the development of the "Four Great Schools" of the Jin and Yuan dynasties mentioned in Chapter Four and should serve as a warning that the totality of traditional Oriental medicine has been lost. Some of the missing parts have been kept alive by acupuncture traditions other than LA and TCM, such as the various Korean, Japanese and French styles of practice which each emphasize a slightly different etiological factor. This assertion merits more extensive treatment than is possible in the context of this work.

8. DEMONIC POSSESSION. One of the more striking differences between LA and TCM is in their handling of the subject of demonology. Demons constitute an etiological category which has been discussed in Chinese medical writings extending at least throughout China's entire dynastic history. As pointed out in Unschuld-1, demonology formed an earlier stratum of medical though in China than did the systematic correspondence theories of Yin Yang and the Five Elements, which added a new layer of medical thought rather than replacing the earlier one. In Chapter Four of the text I have presented the hypothesis that acupuncture itself most likely originated from the exorcistic practices of the early shamans or wu. In Chen Yen's tripartite etiological model, demonic possession belonged in the miscellaneous category, meaning it was neither an exogenous nor an endogenous cause of disease, strictly speaking, and Zhang Jiebing enumerated demonology as the thirteenth medical specialty in his 1624 work, the *Classic of Categories* (Unschuld-1, p. 220). TCM, in adopting a materialist framework, naturally rejected the demonological aspects of traditional Chinese medical thought as mere superstition. LA, on the other hand, retained the category of demonic possession, indicating by this term a loss of control over one's own energy or life-force, and interestingly, LA recapitulates the historical record by considering such possession to be a "block" which must be treated prior to applying Five Element or systematic correspondence types of acupuncture. See also the entry on Seven Dragons for Seven Devils.

9. AGGRESSIVE ENERGY. Like Demonic Possession, the term Aggressive Energy or AE exists in LA parlance, but not in TCM. Like Possession, AE constitutes a "block" precluding Five Element acupuncture treatment, and is considered a foreign type of energy that has become mixed in with the individual's own normal energy. In Chapter Five I discussed the concept of AE and established that this term was coined by Jacques Lavier, one of Worsley's teachers as a translation of the Chinese term xie qi (邪氣) more commonly translated as Perverse or Evil Qi (Lavier-3, pps. 155-164). Lavier's unique teachings about xie qi apparently derive from an oral tradition in Taiwan based on the teachings of Liu Wan-su, who proposed that ultimately all forms of xie qi would transform to Fire. Lavier mentioned two methods of draining xie qi, only one of which was incorporated into LA. This method involves needling the Back Shu Points (called Associated Effect Points in LA) of the Zang Organs involved, and retaining the needles until all traces of erythema (Fire) have dissipated. Lavier's second method involved draining xie qi from the Five Shu Points (Five Element Points in LA). While TCM does not describe Aggressive Energy as such, it does make an important distinction between Normal (Zheng Qi 正氣) and Perverse (Xie Qi 邪氣) Energy. See the next entry for the different conceptions of Zheng and Xie Qi in LA and TCM.

10. THE NATURE OF EXCESS AND DEFICIENCY. TCM stipulates that Excess (shi 實) refers to the state of preponderance of pathogenic factors (xie qi) while Deficiency (xu 虛) refers to the state of insufficiency of normal resistance (zheng qi 正氣), so in TCM these terms are not commensurate (*Essentials*, p. 63). The closest parallel to this conceptualization in LA is that of Aggressive Energy (AE) which is something to be eliminated from the human body. What remains behind is considered to be Normal Energy, which may be Excess in certain Organs and Meridians, and simultaneously Deficient in others. In this second conceptualization of Excess and Deficiency, the two terms both refer to Normal Energy (hyperfunctioning and hypofunctioning), and are therefore commensurate. The primary treatment strategy in LA is thus to redistribute Energy from sites of Excess to those of Deficiency, rather than to drain or disperse it. These different interpretations of the pathological states of Excess and Deficiency are thus responsible for the radically different approaches to treatment found in TCM and LA. The only explicit discussion of these two different concepts of Excess and Deficiency in the Oriental literature, of which I am aware, occurs in Fukushima's text, page 161, however it is likely that many further examples will turn up when a more significant percentage of the voluminous Oriental medical corpus has been translated. Other Japanese sources (e.g. Ohsawa-1, pp. 74-75) reflect an implicit understanding of this second concept of Excess and Deficiency (again reflecting the Japanese influence on LA, primarily through Schmidt, Munster and Ono) although it is also present, for example, in Soulié de Morant -1, p. 66.

11. HUSBAND-WIFE IMBALANCES. LA posits three major types of "block" or pathological states that must be treated before employing its more typical Five Element approach to treatment based on identification of the Causative Factor (see entry below). The first two types of "block" are Demonic Possession and Aggressive Energy, both of which have already been described as pathological states in which some "outside factor" is disrupting normal functioning. The third type of "block" is called a Husband-Wife imbalance (H/W), and it reflects a situation where the abnormal distribution of Excesses and Deficiencies of Normal Energy has created a breakdown in the operation of the very laws of nature (Yin Yang and Five Element) which sustain life. Thus the H/W is considered a fatal type of pathology if left untreated. An H/W is diagnosed when pulses on the left wrist are weaker overall than those on the right wrist, although it is said that the more important difference between the pulses on the two sides is qualitative rather than quantitative—the left side pulses being of poorer quality overall than the right side pulses. In traditional Chinese thought the left side is Yang (and therefore male) while the right side is Yin (and therefore female), and Chinese family life is markedly paternalistic, so this idea would seem self-evident to Chinese practitioners. Its first mention in the Western literature was in Soulié de Morant-2 (Volume II, Chapter VIII) where the following quotation from "Iang Ko-sienn" is given: "Weak husband, strong wife—thus there is destruction. Strong husband, weak wife—thus there is security. Ta Tch III p. 32V" Soulié de Morant did not advocate a specific protocol for treating this imbalance, but his close grouping of the Laws of Husband-Wife, Mother-Son and Midday-Midnight was clearly the original basis for the incorporation of these laws into LA, following their translation into English in Mann-1, pps. 101-107.

12. THE LAW OF MIDDAY-MIDNIGHT. In his chart of the Five Elements, Worsley cites this law immediately after that of Husband-Wife, just as had Mann. Soulié de Morant presented them in the opposite order, so it is easy to trace the line of thought from Soulié de Morant to Mann to Worsley. Neither Soulié de Morant nor Mann cited any classical references for this law, however, the Chinese Organ clock on which it is based is universally recognized in Oriental medicine—only the details of how to apply it vary. In essence it states that each Organ has a two hour time period during which it is most active, and an opposite two hour period twelve hours later during which it is least active. One might suspect pathology in one of the correlated Organs, at its zenith or nadir of activity, if a symptom recurs regularly at a given time. Midday-Midnight is a translation of Zi Wu (子 午) which are the names (Earthly Branches) of the time periods from 11 p.m. to 1 a.m. and from 11 a.m. to 1 p.m. This term also appears in the phrase "zi wu liu zhu fa" which refers to biorhythmic methodology in general, and was probably what Soulié de Morant translated as "Law of Midday-Midnight." Biorhythmic methods were a development of the theory of phase energetics cited in Chapter Four as becoming an important aspect of acupuncture theory at least as early as the Tang dynasty. Various Chinese and European traditions include protocols for using the Law of Midday-Midnight in formulating acupuncture treatments, but perhaps because these are based on balancing Yin and Yang rather than the Five Elements, they were not incorporated into LA. The influence of this law on LA is found, however, in the use of Horary Points and the Four Needle technique which will be discussed in separate entries.

13. ENTRY-EXIT BLOCK. I stated earlier that in LA there are three major types of block which preclude Five Element treatment: Possession, AE and H/W. In addition, there are "minor" types of blockage of the flow of Energy which may interfere with the efficacy of Five Element treatment, although they do not in themselves lead to progressive deterioration or fatality if ignored—at worst they seem to dampen the efficacy of treatment, so that it may only be partially successful. The main example of this kind of block is called an Entry-Exit block. It is felt to represent a failure of communication or Energy flow from one Meridian to the next Meridian following the superficial or Wei circulation. There is no specific dogma concerning the etiology of Entry-Exit blocks, although the most commonly diagnosed one in LA, between the Liver and Lung Meridians, is frequently seen in patients who take medications that are detoxified or metabolized by the liver. These blocks are diagnosed by persistent imbalances on the pulse between two Organs that follow sequentially in the superficial circulation, in spite of seemingly appropriate treatment to harmonize them. A special class of Points called Entry Points and Exit Points is employed in treating such blocks. Although these Points are not mentioned in any English language TCM texts, their use was taught to Radha Thambirajah at the Shanghai Military Medical College in the 1960's, and is also part of the Daoist lineage taught to Jeffrey Yuen. Their initial description in the West was in Niboyet-2 where they were associated with the biorhythmic methods or Zi Wu Liu Zhu Fa mentioned in the previous entry. Niboyet learned this approach from his unnamed Chinese teacher, and in turn was the source for its description in Mann-1, whence its incorporation into LA. Another type of "minor" block is that between or at the specific levels of Body, Mind and Spirit, which will be described in a separate entry.

14. THE LAW OF CURE. This dictum, a component of the LA syllabus, states that in the natural course of healing, patients may experience a recurrence of previous symptoms in a characteristic order—from deeper to more superficial, from above to below, from more vital to less vital Organs, and in the reverse order of their original appearance. There is no mention of the Law of Cure in TCM, as this law was formulated by the German-American physician, Constantin Hering, one of the guiding lights of homeopathic medicine in the nineteenth century. One may well ask how it became incorporated into the teachings of a school of traditional acupuncture. As recounted in Chapter Five, the original proponents of acupuncture in France, notably Soulié de Morant and de La Fuÿe were intrigued by the similarities between acupuncture and homeopathy, and actively tried to integrate them. Many of the later pioneers of acupuncture in England also had previous training in various branches of what is now called complementary medicine, including physiotherapy, naturopathy, osteopathy, herbalism and homeopathy. In fact, Worsley's closest associate, at the time he founded his own college and formulated LA, was a homeopath, Malcolm Stemp. Other early faculty members were also trained in homeopathy, including Dick Van Buren who subsequently founded his own acupuncture college. At some point, their homeopathic convictions found their way into the Leamington syllabus. A related naturopathic principle, known as the healing crisis, is also taught as part of LA, but in this case the concept is frequently mentioned by Oriental practitioners, although it is not usually written about, and is not mentioned in TCM texts. A healing crisis involves a temporary, usually short-lived episode following treatment during which the presenting symptoms are increased in severity, following which they markedly decrease in severity for a more prolonged period. This phenomenon is commonly described by the saying, "You've got to get worse before you get better." It was enunciated as a universal finding by Yoshimasu Todo in Japan during the eighteenth century (Ozaki, pps. 218-224), but in this case I would attribute its presence in LA as due to parallel development rather than to transmission of doctrine from Japan to England.

15. COLOR, SOUND, ODOR AND EMOTION. Traditionally, examination of a patient comprised four components: seeing, hearing (plus smelling) questioning and feeling. While all surviving traditions acknowledge this paradigm, they put it into practice with marked differences in emphasis and interpretation. In TCM for example, the main examination skills include observing the tongue, feeling the pulse, and eliciting the patient's history in a ritualized manned based on Zhang Jie-bin's "Song of the Ten Questions." LA emphasizes its own set of examination skills which are described in the following four entries. The first one, "Color, sound, odor and emotion" is a mnemonic phrase used to remind the practitioner of the essential components of a Five Element diagnosis. Each of these four perceptual categories has five possible findings, so as to correlate with the Five Elements. This is admittedly an oversimplification, as there are, for example, many more than five colors that can be seen in examining patients, however, these can all be classified as subcategories of one of the five basic colors: red (or lack thereof), yellow, white, blue and green. The subcategories (for example, a yellowish shade of green) are interpreted as reflecting a deeper level of diagnosis, the Element within the Element (Earth within Wood in this case) to be described in a separate entry. Before elaborating on the details of how one determines the specific color, sound, odor and emotion present in a clinical setting, I should mention that these findings are the basis for diagnosing the Causative Factor or CF, which is also described in a separate entry.

The five colors may be seen on the patient's face, principally on the temples and secondarily under the eyes, on the smile creases and around the mouth. These colors are subtle emanations, and not the frank skin tone we normally observe. Being energetic signals, the characteristic colors should intensify and fade as the patient fluctuates from moment to moment in the degree of stress on his major Elemental imbalance during the course of the examination—particularly the questioning phase. The associations of the colors with the Elements are standard throughout TOM with the following exceptions: Wood is associated with green in LA, but may be associated with either green or blue in other traditions. The original Chinese word qing (青) includes both these colors, and some modern translators have chosen the term cyan to reflect this ambiguity. The other disputed color is the one associated with the Water Element. Most references specify black in contrast to the blue chosen in LA. Matsumoto and Birch, on page 96, in describing the Japanese Meridian Therapy tradition, note that both blue and black are associated with the Water Element which they ascribe to a reference in the *Su Wen*. In Ni's translation of the *Su Wen*, Chapter 72 describes "a deep blue energy emanating from solid kidneys to the north." Matsumoto and Birch also confirm many of the facial areas in which to notice these colors, as specified in LA, thus it is likely that this component of LA derives from Worsley's Japanese sources previously cited.

The five sounds (specified in *Su Wen* Chapter 5) are shouting, laughing, singing, weeping and groaning, although there is considerable variation between different translators—true also for the odors and emo-

tions. Like the five colors, these are all normal components of the fluctu-
ating pattern of healthy speech, but under stress, the sound associated with
the imbalanced Element becomes predominant. In a similar manner, the
odor associated with the imbalanced Element (specified in *Su Wen* Chapter
4), also predominates, being either rancid, scorched, fragrant, rotten or
putrid. Finally, the same is true for the associated emotion (specified in *Su
Wen* Chapter 5) which in LA dogma would be anger, joy (or lack thereof),
sympathy, grief or fear. The only major disagreement between LA dogma
and other traditional schools would be in the emotion associated with the
Earth Element. In LA it is sympathy, while in most other references it is
given as a variation of either pensiveness or worry (Lu, p. 37; Matsumoto
and Birch, p. 98; Hashimoto-1, p. 39). We can see how sympathy became
enshrined in LA dogma by noting that prior authors who adopted this
translation from the *Su Wen* included Veith (p. 119) originally and Mann-
1 (p. 94) subsequently (presumably guided by Veith's choice). Perusing the
Five Element chart given by Mann, his text seems clearly to be the source
for the terminology of color, sound, odor and emotion used in LA, much as
it was the source for the various "Laws of the Five Elements" previously discussed. What is unique about LA in this regard is not the terminology, but
the process by which these concepts are engaged. Although this process will
be discussed under a separate entry as rapport, I will give a brief description
of its application to the examination in what has become known as "emotion testing." In order to bring out the patient's color, sound, odor and
emotion most clearly, the Element responsible must be under some degree
of stress. This can be accomplished as the practitioner, while interacting
with the patient during the interview and examination, creates emotional-
ly challenging moments, and keenly observes the patient's reactions.
"Emotion testing" harkens back to Zhu Zhen-heng's "living noose" style of
treatment mentioned in Chapter Four, and suggests that Worsley's methodology owes as much to his Chinese teachers as it does to those from Japan.

16. THE RADIAL PULSES. As described in Chapter Four, the assignments of Organs and Meridians to the twelve radial pulse positions differ
in LA and TCM. These differences are summarized in Figure 63, which
points out that the LA schema is based on the *Nan Jing*, considered to be of
highest authority in the Japanese Five Element tradition. These Japanese
schools are commonly referred to under two different names, the first being
Meridian Therapy (Keiraku Chiryo) and the second being Pulse Diagnosis
(Myakushin). In comparing methodologies, it is clear that the examination of the pulse in LA is Japanese in derivation. Unlike the Chinese procedure adopted in TCM, in LA the pulses are felt with the tips rather than
the pads of the fingers applied perpendicularly as illustrated in Figure 126.
This methodology was transmitted to Europe by Masae Hashimoto, whose
clinical skills were then propagated by George Ohsawa, Heribert Schmidt,
and Elza Munster. Worsley could have become acquainted with it through
either Schmidt or Munster or another Myakushin teacher such as Ono.
Another feature of the LA pulse examination that appears to be Japanese in

origin is the procedure for classifying each of the twelve radial pulses by a "plus" or "minus" to designate its relative state of Excess or Deficiency. This methodology is described in Ohsawa-1 (p. 51) and was presumably reflective of Hashimoto's teaching, of which Ohsawa's writing is a record. A similar system for recording the gradations of Deficiency and Excess numerically on a scale from one to eight was described in Lawson-Wood (p. 26) whose book was written close to the time of his initial contact with Ohsawa (although this contact was reported as having begun the year after the book was written) and before his association with Worsley. Since this methodology is absent from the works of de La Fuÿe and Stiefvater (as far as I know) who were Lawson-Wood's other sources, the most likely lineage would be through Ohsawa. The issue of establishing the origin of this system of recording pulses, which is part of LA, is important, because it is a necessary precondition for using the transfer methodology in treatment, a topic of great contention and mysterious lineage to be discussed in a subsequent entry.

17. EXAMINATION OF THE ABDOMEN.   Although LA does not employ examination of the tongue, which plays such an important role in TCM, it does make use of two procedures which occupy an equally important place in Japanese traditions, but are conversely less important in TCM. The first of these is examination of the abdomen, or Fukushin, also known as Hara diagnosis (Matsumoto and Birch, pps. 46-47).   Originally a Chinese idea mentioned in the *Nan Jing* (Chapters 16 and 56), it later flowered in Japan where numerous methodologies and interpretations were developed by practitioners of both the herbal Kampo and acupuncture traditions. In examining the abdomen, different areas are associated with the various Organs and palpatory findings correlate to their associated Organs. The locations on the abdomen in LA which correspond to the various Organs are essentially the same as those taught in Meridian Therapy, and are based on the *Nan Jing*. Hashimoto and Schmidt were largely responsible for introducing this procedure in Europe.

18. THE AKABANE TEST.   Perhaps the clearest evidence that the style of acupuncture I have designated as LA could not possibly be identical to that practiced in antiquity, as its founder has claimed, is its inclusion of the Akabane Test, a procedure named after the twentieth century Japanese practitioner who devised it.   The test uses a burning stick of incense to test the patient's heat sensitivity at the terminal nail points of the Meridians, for symmetry between the left and right sides. Any asymmetry found indicates an imbalance or malfunction of the associated Meridian or Organ, and can be corrected by one of several treatment protocols. LA specifies the treatment of choice as tonification of the Luo or Connecting Point of the involved Meridian on the deficient side (i.e., the side less sensitive to heat). The test was developed by Akabane Kobe (see Figure 158) one of the numerous practitioners Schmidt met in Japan, and whose works Schmidt publicized in Europe. The inclusion of the Akabane Test in LA is one of the more compelling arguments for identifying Schmidt as the German physician who had strongly influenced Worsley's thinking. Worsley was fascinated with the Akabane Test, and there were a number of occasions when the author observed Worsley predicting in advance which Meridians in a given patient would exhibit an Akabane imbalance, and on which side they would be deficient. Although Worsley gave no explanation for how he did this, the most likely explanation would appear to be that he was perceiving asymmetries in the Elemental colors on the two sides. The existence of imbalances between the left and right halves of a single Meridian had been described prior to the discovery of the Akabane Test, and in Niboyet-2, pages 68 to 71, their identification by pulse diagnosis is explained in detail.

19. The Causative Factor. Having ascertained that LA was developed syncretically from many sources, it should not be surprising that the component teachings of LA have themselves evolved over time. Thus, based on interviews with a number of Worsley's early students from the U.S. and U.K., it appears to the author that the notion of the Causative Factor was one of LA's more recent developments. The Causative Factor, or CF, is now the basic diagnostic finding in LA, specifying the Element or Official which will receive the most attention in the formulation of acupuncture treatment for each patient. In the earliest days, the conceptualization of diagnosis seems to have been the least developed aspect of LA. In those early days, treatment was aimed at rebalancing the patient's energy based on the color, sound, odor, emotion and pulse findings, but there was initially no presumption that all of these findings on examination would point to one Element or Official—indeed it was common for examination findings to point to two, three or more different Elements. With the introduction of the concept of the CF, there has been a gradual tendency for LA examinations to show more coherency around a single Elemental imbalance. The technical definition of the CF is that it is the Element or Official whose chronic state of imbalance can not be completely corrected by nature itself, and which in turn is responsible for producing or at least allowing imbalances to develop and persist in the other Elements or Officials. The CF thus becomes the primary focus for acupuncture treatment. A pragmatic rule for identifying the CF was developed by one of Worsley's American students, Jim McCormick, a rule which he called the "three legs of the stool." By this rule, at least three findings from color, sound, odor and emotion should point to the same Element in order to establish it as the CF. This rule is not without exceptions, the author having observed Worsley himself deciding on a CF with less than three corroborating legs, and in one case identifying a CF in a patient who had no "legs" at all associated with the CF! These latter cases are, however, the exception rather than the rule, but they do indicate that perhaps the concept of the CF still awaits a clearer articulation. While TCM has no concept strictly paralleling that of the CF (although its syndromes do most commonly focus on one Organ), other traditions with a more predominant Five Element basis do. Thus, the various schools of Meridian Therapy in

Japan and the Korean Constitutional style of acupuncture all specify a particular Element and Organ as the focus of treatment for each patient based on Five Element considerations, although they differ in regard to beliefs about when this predominant imbalance becomes established in life, and how invariant or changeable it may be over time. LA does not establish any dogma about when the CF originates, although it is almost always determined before childhood is over, and does not change over time (Worsley-3, pps. 29-30). Fukushima employs the concept of akashi in a manner that closely parallels the notion of CF, but in the case histories cited in his book, the akashi does occasionally change over time. For Honma, constitutional types, a parallel concept, were fixed, and in the Korean Constitutional Acupuncture style taught by Kuon Dowon, the constitutional types are not only fixed, but genetically inborn. The question of constitutional types has a very long history of discussion in Oriental medicine and was originally mentioned as early as the *Nei Jing* (*Ling Shu*, Chapter 64). As a final comment on Worsley's inclusion of the concept of the CF in LA, I should once again mention the occurrence of this term in the writings of the Protestant missionary W.R. Morse, who also mentioned the Five Elements, the Officials and the phrase "Body, Mind and Spirit," each of which appears as an entry in this appendix. It would not be surprising, therefore, if Worsley took some inspiration from Morse in formulating his concept of the CF.

20. ELEMENT WITHIN ELEMENT. To a first approximation, the identification of the CF establishes the diagnosis in LA. There are, however, two further levels of diagnostic specificity that can be useful in understanding the symptomatology, and in choosing the most appropriate treatment. The first of these is called "the Element within." Each of the Five Elements is conceptualized as itself being composed in turn of all of the Five Elements, so for example, Wood is composed of Wood, Fire, Earth, Metal and Water. This level is called the Element within the Element. Thus, a patient diagnosed as a Wood CF might be further diagnosed as having Fire within, meaning the Fire is out of balance within the Wood. The basis for diagnosing the Element within is the same as for diagnosing the CF—it is reflected in the patient's color, sound, odor and emotion. According to Worsley, the Element within causes a shading of the predominant color, sound, odor and emotion rather than a second distinct color, sound, odor and emotion. Thus in a Wood CF, Fire within, the green color would be a slightly reddish green, the odor would be a slightly scorched type of rancid, etc. The element within is itself in turn composed of each of the Five Elements, and in LA, diagnoses are formally specified to this third level: Element within Element within Element. For example in the previous case the complete Elemental diagnosis might be Earth within Fire within Wood—meaning Wood CF (primary), Fire within (secondary) and Earth within that (tertiary). Again the process for determining the tertiary diagnosis is analogously based on color, sound, odor and emotion. Without going into details, it is easy to see that the secondary level, or Element within, has a physical correlate in the Meridian system: Each Meridian corresponds to one Element, and also has a Point for each of the Five Elements along its trajectory. Thus the Liver and Gallbladder Meridians corresponding to our hypothetical Wood CF each have Fire Points (the Element within), Liver-2 and Gallbladder-38, that might be the most effective Points to employ at a given stage in this patient's treatment using the Element within Element approach, which is an advanced level of treatment technique in LA. Some strategies for employing the concept of Element within Element, based on passages in the *Nei Jing* and *Nan Jing*, can be found in the article by Leung, and this issue is frequently alluded to in the various schools of Meridian Therapy. Strategies for employing the tertiary level of Elemental diagnosis have not as yet been articulated, as far as I know.

21. BODY, MIND AND SPIRIT. The second type of further diagnostic specificity in LA relates not to the Elements, but to the level of Body, Mind or Spirit that is the focus of the patient's imbalance. Bodily imbalances are usually the result of simple physical trauma—a sprained ankle for example. Mental and Spiritual imbalances can also present with physical complaints that can mimic Bodily imbalances, as for example in many cases of arthritis of the ankle. The distinction is not in the nature of the symptom, but in the underlying cause which can only be discovered by a holistic evaluation of the patient's overall state of health—is their thinking appropriate and coherent on the Mental level, and are their values and goals those of someone in balance with themselves, their family, society and their environment on the Spiritual level? The diagnosis of the level involved has implications not only for understanding the severity of the patient's illness (prognosis) but also in the choice of treatment strategies. Certain Points have more powerful effects on the Mental level while others act more powerfully on the Spiritual level (see the entry on Spirit of the Points). While the terminology of Body, Mind and Spirit would appear to reflect the influence on Worsley of Western authors such as Morse, it also appears in the quotation from Ohsawa cited previously, "You can determine the stage or depth of the illness, evaluate the degree of physical, physiological, mental or spiritual disease. This latter category of illness is the hardest to cure, but unfortunately it's very widespread. Spiritual blindness is a much worse affliction than mere physical blindness." (Ohsawa-1, p. 38). One might add that in fact spiritual blindness can be the cause of physical blindness. LA, in its emphasis on diagnosing the Elemental imbalance (CF) and level (Body, Mind or Spirit), employs a non-symptomatic approach to diagnosis (reflected in a non-symptomatic approach to treatment as well). Thus blindness, for example, tells us no more about the essential diagnosis (CF, level) than would a swollen painful ankle. Both complaints might even be expressions of an identical diagnosis! Similar non-symptomatic approaches to diagnosis and treatment were described by both Bach in the Western literature, and by Ohsawa who wrote that, "One should never try to simply eliminate (the patient's) suffering, pain or other symptoms. . . . Symptomatic treatment is actually complicity in the original violation of natural law which was responsible for the problem in the first place." (Ohsawa-1, p. 92). Ohsawa's comments reflect the impact of Shinto and Daoist lineages on LA.

22. ENERGY TRANSFERS. It is only in the realm of treatment that the tenets of LA become relatively more objective that subjective. Thus the exact location of a Point, the state of the pulses, the identity of the CF and the level affected in a given patient may all be open to disagreement between practitioners, but given a specific pulse pattern there are clear-cut treatment protocols in LA that will help to restore balance, even if the CF and level are unknown. These protocols in fact formed the basis for treatment in LA prior to the development of the concept of the CF. For this reason I have called these rules for achieving balance by transferring energy, the "central dogma" of LA. Curiously, this most objective component of LA is the one with the least clearly articulated historical precedent. Even as early as the *Nei Jing*, the concept of transferring energy from where it is Excess to where it is Deficient is clearly implicated (e.g. Ni's interpretive translation of *Su Wen* Chapter 5 states, "If there is a qi deficiency in a particular location or channel, the qi can be conducted or guided from other channels to supplement the weakness," while Lu's more literal translation simply reads, "energy deficiency should be treated by the energy induced from other regions"), however none of the early classics described any specific methods for carrying out these transfers. The use of energy transfers depends on knowledge of both the Five Element cycles of Creation and Control, and the Command Points of each Meridian. The Five Element cycles are described and illustrated in Chapter Two and operate via Secondary Vessels as indicated in entry No. 4 of this appendix. The Command Points constitute that category of Points with predictable actions on the energy balance within and between Meridians, and includes the Tonification and Sedation Points as special cases of the Five Element Points, the Source Points, the Connecting (Luo) Points, the Alarm (Front Collecting or Mo) Points, the Associated Effect (Back Shu) Points, and the Entry and Exit Points. The concept of Command Points, so crucial to an understanding of energy transfer strategies, was apparently first mentioned in the West in Niboyet-1, p. 167 (1951). Niboyet's source for these aspects of his teachings (not derived from Soulié de Morant) was an anonymous Chinese instructor, and although no definitive lineage can be established for the various energy transfer protocols, they do appear to be Chinese in origin. The British College of Acupuncture with Worsley as Chairman, taught this methodology from its inception, i.e., before Worsley's first visit to the Orient (it is mentioned in the Acupuncture Association Newsletter, July 1965) and as such it represents an early stratum of the material which later became incorporated in LA. The most obvious source for the presence of these teachings in the BCA would be Jacques Lavier, who taught Worsley along with most of the other BCA faculty members in 1963. Lavier published some details of energy transfers via the Five Elements in his translation of Wu Wei-p'ing's textbook, but I have been unable to corroborate any of the various hypotheses for where he had learned this material, including his own claim of its Taiwanese origin. I have indicated in the text my reasons for favoring the hypothesis of Ed Wong from Singapore as his most likely Oriental source. Two other treatment strategies, the use of Horary Points and the Four Needle technique, point to earlier methods based upon which the idea of transfers might have developed. Horary Points are the Points on a given Meridian that correspond to its own associated Element, especially when used during its associated (two hour) time period. These Points which are commonly used in LA are associated with the biorhythmic (zi wu liu zhu fa) and phase energetic (wu yun liu qi) schools of Chinese medicine, which started at least as early as the Tang dynasty. Important contributors to these schools of thought, whose work laid a foundation upon which energy transfer methods could have been developed, would include Dou Han-qing and his son Dou Gui-fang (who described the use of the Five Element Points in phase energetics), Hua Shou (who described the open and closed times of the Command Points in biorhythmic treatment) and finally, Xu Feng and Gao Wu (who developed the concept of Tonificiation and Sedation Points as special cases of the Five Element Points). The Four Needle technique, while employing Horary Points and effectively though indirectly transferring energy, is derived from a different acupuncture tradition having been proposed initially by a Korean Buddhist monk, Sa Am, in the 1600's. Conceptually, it strengthens Deficient Meridians and sedates Excess Meridians directly, although the new state of balance it engenders can be thought of as equivalent to an energy transfer. In keeping with its disparate origin, it entered LA not through Lavier, but via the published work of Mann. The Four Needle technique is still commonly used by practitioners in Japan and Korea as a repeated protocol for "root" treatment, while the transfer treatments used in LA are generally not repeated, since the pulse pattern upon which LA treatment is based is felt to be much more variable from session to session than it is in these other styles. Worsley adapted the Four Needle technique for use in LA in the special circumstance of a Husband-Wife imbalance, in which case it can be repeated until the H/W is broken. Future investigators are cautioned to clearly distinguish the conceptual differences between energy transfer strategies and those akin to the Four Needle technique in trying to further elucidate the origin of the former. The logical place to look for some mention of transfers would be in the *Great Compendium* of Yang Ji-zhou which has not been translated into English yet. The only definite mention, with specific examples, of energy transfers in the Oriental literature of which I am aware is in the book by Fukushima (p. 161) where the Chinese term "shu" is used—the same term which is the collective name for the Five Element Points, and is more commonly translated as "transport." Fukushima describes transfers in the same sense as in LA, meaning a technique that is applied to a Deficient Meridian to attract energy to it from an Excess Meridian. The examples he gives include treating coupled Meridians and those in Control cycle relationships. One final point about the transfer protocols, is that there is no universal agreement among the various sources that describe them. The most common areas of difference concern the manner of use of the Connecting (Luo) Points and the Points to transfer energy via the Control cycle, while everyone seems to agree on the protocol to transfer energy via the Creative cycle. The whole subject is far too complex for a thorough presentation here, but the basic protocols employed in LA are as follows:

a) When the coupled Meridians of the same Element are out of balance with each other, tonify the Connecting Point of the Deficient Meridian.

b) When two Meridians along the Creative Cycle are out of balance, and the Mother Meridian is Excess with respect to the Child Meridian, tonify the Mother Point (Tonification Point) of the Child Meridian. Both Meridians must be of the same (Yin-Yang) polarity.

c) When two Meridians along the Control cycle are out of balance, and the Controlling Meridian is Excess with respect to the Controlled Meridian, tonify the Controlling Point of the Controlled Meridian. This protocol only works for the Yin Meridians.

The common aspect of these three protocols is needling the Deficient Meridian to attract energy from the Excess Meridian.

23. SPIRIT OF THE POINTS. Each acupuncture Point has one or more traditional names which are purported to be emblems of their individual esoteric therapeutic potentials. This aspect of traditional teaching can be used to select Points to best match the level of imbalance. For example, some Points such as the group called "Windows of the Sky" are preferentially indicated in Spirit level imbalances because they all contain the term "Sky" or "Heaven" (tian) which is related to Spirit in Chinese metaphysics. The "Windows of the Sky" were originally mentioned in *Ling Shu* Chapters Two, Five and Twenty One, and found their way into LA from Mann-1, pps. 133-134. Like the doctrine of the Officials, the Spirit of the Points involves a kind of personification of components of the human microcosm. This Point personification was an important development of the medically inclined religious Daoists, and is exemplified in the *Yellow Court Classic* (c. second century) a component of the *Daoist Patrology (Dao Zang).* Contemporary Daoist practitioners such as Jeffrey Yuen in New York make extensive use of the Spirit of the Points in teaching and practicing acupuncture. Worsley's inclusion of this concept in LA most likely reflects the influence of Lavier, who gave multiple examples of how to choose Points based on their traditional names in his 1966 work (pps. 245-248).

24. SEVEN DRAGONS FOR SEVEN DEVILS. This picturesque phrase is the name for a formulaic protocol for treating cases of demonic possession due to either External Devils (GV 20, B 11, B 23, B 61) or Internal Devils (CV 15 or the Master Point halfway from CV 15 to CV 14, S 25, S 32, S 41). Worsley claimed to have learned this treatment from his "Master Hsiue." Historically, a similar protocol called the Thirteen Ghost Points was used by Sun Si-miao in the Tang dynasty. The Internal Dragons treatment, including the Master Point on the conception Vessel was identified as a Tang dynasty prescription for hysteria by an aged acupuncturist interviewed by Allegra Wint at the Yunnan College of TCM in Kunming in 1982 (personal communication from Ms. Wint).

25. NEEDLE TECHNIQUE. LA employs a considerably different needle technique than is typical of TCM. The goal of TCM acupuncture is for the patient to experience a sensation called "de Qi," which can be perceived as heaviness, soreness, aching or distention. In LA on the other hand, it is the practitioner who feels the "Qi" through the handle of the needle, and it is not considered necessary for the patient to feel anything at all. Worsley's clinical nickname, "the Feather," undoubtedly refers to this delicacy of touch. This aspect of LA needle technique is shared with the majority of Japanese styles of practice, to which Worsley was exposed. A second aspect of LA needle technique which distinguishes it from TCM is the rapidity of needling in tonification, a procedure which is accomplished in a few seconds. Again, this echoes the practice in many Japanese styles (see Ohsawa-1, p. 258). It was also the technique taught by Lavier which would have prepared the way for Worsley's subsequent Japanese teachers. In both of these styles antecedent to LA, sedation or dispersion is accomplished by a more prolonged retention of the needle, from twenty to thirty minutes being typical.

26. RAPPORT. Successful treatment in any medical system depends on many factors including the intangible doctor-patient relationship. Thus, rapport between practitioner and patient is important in TCM as well as in LA, but in the latter approach it has added significance. Unlike training in TCM, in LA the single clinical skill which receives the most time and attention is learning to develop one's rapport with individual patients. In my mind there is no question that this harkens back to LA's roots in shamanistic practices. Also, it is only when rapport is achieved that the patient's true identity—not only persona, but also color, sound, odor and emotion—will reveal themselves behind the habitual social mask. Thus, the practitioner must join with the patient in a vision of themselves, not only as they are at the moment, but as they would be if they were totally healthy in Body, Mind and Spirit. This ideal is based on the practitioner as educator, and is firmly rooted in the *Nei Jing*. It also calls on the practitioner to himself embody the highest standards of knowledge, skill, wisdom, compassion and humility. In the words of Christoph Hufeland (see Fig.111) presaging a virtually identical statement by J.R. Worsley some two hundred years later, "Never forget that it is not you but only Nature who can heal disease. You are only an assistant who increases Nature's capacity and performance."*

---

*Hufeland's quotation is cited in McGavack, p. 15. Compare it to the following from Worsley-5, p. xi: "Only Nature can cure disease. Practitioners only assist Nature, acting as instruments of Nature in putting the patient back on the path to health."

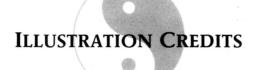

ILLUSTRATION CREDITS

LISTED BY FIGURE NUMBER

Neal White: frontispiece, 17, 23, 32, 50, 52, 53, 55, 140A
Pedro Chan: 1
Tobe Soshichiro: 2, 10, 78, 119, 120, 129, 130, 132, 141, 142, 143, 150,
    151, 152, 153, 155, 157, 158, 159, 160, 177, 184B, 187, 204, 205,
    209, 216, 217
Traditional Acupuncture Society: 4, 35, 36, 37, 193
Xinhua News Agency: 5
Sally Reston and The New York Times: 6
People's Medical Publishing House: 15, 16
Yul-Hwa-Dang: 24
British Museum, London: 25
National Museum, Tokyo: 26
Foreign Languages Press: 27
Chengdu College of TCM: 28
United Features Syndicate: 30
China Welfare Institute: 33
Sheng-chi t'u: 34
National Museum of Korea: 39
Joseph Needham: 40, 212
Oriental Healing Arts Institute: 41, 57, 59, 72, 73, 77, 93, 95, 161, 174
China Books: 42, 62, 64, 68
Seligman Collection: 43
Alan Covell: 44, 45, 46
Editions Payot: 47
Jon Covell: 48, 49
Wellcome Institute for the History of Medicine: 54
Wolfram Eberhard: 56
National Palace Museum, Taipei: 58, 62
Johns Hopkins Press: 60
Hamard Foundation: 61, 65, 66, 70, 71, 74, 75, 76, 79, 81, 82, 83, 84,
    85, 87, 88, 89
University of California, San Francisco: 67
K. Chimin Wong and Wu Lien-Teh: 69, 122
Blue Poppy Press: 86
Lok Yee-Kung: 90
Wu Liu: 91A
Stephan Palos: 91B
Ren Jianning: 92
Gillian Foulkes: 94, 195, 196
John Worsley: 96, 97, 98, 99, 100, 101, 102, 166, 176, 207
Robert Felt: 103
Harry Cadman: 104
Joyce Lawson-Wood: 105
Royston Low: 106, 107

Peter Firebrace: 108
George Ohsawa Macrobiotic Foundation: 109
Ronald Kotzsch: 110, 115, 116, 215
Frankfurt Goethe Museum: 111
Trevor Cook: 112, 113
East West Journal: 114
Meridiens: 117, 121
Hashimoto Mariko: 118, 125, 126, 127A and B, 128, 131
J.R. Worsley: 123, 181B
Roger De la Fuÿe: 124
Takenouchi Misao: 127C and D
Norman Ozaki: 133, 134, 135, 136, 137, 138
H. Ota: 139
Masaru Toguchi: 140B
Shudo Denmei: 144
Fukushima Kodo: 145
Association Française d'Acupuncture: 146
Mme. J. Schatz: 147, 190, 191
Johannes Bischko: 148
Margaret Ho: 154, 156, 198, 199, 200, 201, 202, 203
Eric Tao: 162
Jean Niboyet-fis: 163
Pat Rose-Neil: 164
Kenneth Basham: 165
Nicholas Sofroniou: 167
G.T. and N.R. Lewith: 168
Philip Chancellor: 169, 170
Denis Lawson-Wood: 171, 172
Mary Austin: 173
Chuang Yu-min: 175
Ryoichi Gunji: 178
Luying Liaw: 179, 181A, 206
Kuon Dowon: 180
Nagayama Toyoko: 182
Anton Jayasuriya: 183
Ralph Luciani: 184A
Radha Thambirajah: 185
A. Duron: 186
Mario Wexu: 188, 189
Nguyen Van Nghi: 192
Jean-Marc Kespi: 194
Eastland Press: 197
Ono Bunkei: 208
W.R. Morse: 213
The Dr. Edward Bach Centre: 214

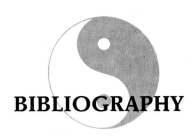

BIBLIOGRAPHY

A Barefoot Doctor's Manual, Running Press, Philadelphia, 1977. Reprinted from U.S. Department of Health, Education and Welfare. Publication number (NIH) 75-695, 1974.

ACTS - *Ancient China's Technology and Science*, compiled by the Institute of the History of Natural Science, Chinese Academy of Sciences. Foreign Languages Press, Beijing, 1983.

Amoyel, J. and M. Wong, "La Médecine Traditionelle Chinoise dans le Monde au XXe Siècle", in *Encyclopédie des Médecines Naturelles*, Paris, 1989.

AOCA - *An Outline of Chinese Acupuncture* compiled by The Academy of Traditional Chinese Medicine, Foreign Languages Press, Peking, 1975.

Artaud, Antonin. *Oeuvres Complètes D'Antonin Artaud*, supplément au Tome 1, Gallimard, Paris, 1970 pps. 127-151 and 224-226.

Austin, Mary. *Acupuncture Therapy*. ASI Publishers, New York, 1972.

Back, Hee Soo, *How To Read Hee Soo Type Electronic Pulse Wave*, Hee Soo Electronic Pulse Institute of Korea, Korea, 1978.

Bancroft, Anne. *Zen*. Thames and Huston, New York, 1979.

Basic Acupuncture Techniques, L. Hsu (trans.) Basic Medicine Books, San Francisco, 1973. Original text by the Editorial Committee for Acupuncture and Moxibustion of the People's Health Publishing House, Beijing, 1964.

Beau, Georges. *La Médecine Chinoise*, Editions du Seuil, France, 1965.

Bensky, Dan, Andrew Gamble and Ted Kaptchuk, *Chinese Herbal Medicine: Materia Medica*, Eastland Press, Seattle, 1986.

Birch, Stephen. "Naming the Unnameable; A Historical Study of Radial Pulse Six Position Diagnosis." Trad. Acup. Soc. J. No. 12. pps. 2-13. 1992.

Bischko, Johannes, *An Introduction to Acupuncture*. Haug Verlag, Heidelberg. 1978.

Bynner, Witter (trans), *The Way of Life According to Lao Tzu*. Capricorn Books, New York. 1962.

Chamfrault, A. *Traité de Médecine Chinoise*; Tome 1, Acupuncture - Moxas - Massages - Saignées. Editions Chamfrault, Angoulême, 1964.

Chamfrault, A. and Nguyen Van Nghi, *Traité de Médecine Chinoise*; Tome VI, L'Energétique Humaine en Médecine Chinoise. La Charente, Angoulême, 1969.

Chan, Pedro. *Acupuncture, Electro-Acupuncture Anaesthesia*. Oriental Trading Co. Los Angeles. 1972.

Chan, Wing-Tsit. *A Source Book in Chinese Philosophy*. Princeton University Press. Princeton. 1963.

Chang, Stephen Thomas. *The Complete Book of Acupuncture*. Celestial Arts. Millbrae, CA 1976.

Chen, Chan-Yuen, *History of Chinese Medical Science Illustrated with Pictures*. Privately published, 1968 (later abridged, revised and edited by Hsu and Peacher - see their entry.)

Cheng Danan-1. *Study of Acupuncture and Moxibustion Therapy*. Public Health Press. Beijing. 1930. (in Chinese)

Cheng Danan-2. *Acupuncture and Moxibusion Study Course.* Public Health Press. Beijing. 1940. (in Chinese)

Cheng Danan-3. *Study of Chinese Acupuncture and Moxibustion.* Public Health Press. Beijing. 1955. (in Chinese)

Cheng, Yen Ping, H. Tan, H.T.Y. Woo and S.H. Chang, *Modern Chinese Acupuncture and Moxibustion.* China Medical College, Tai-Chung. undated.

China's Ancient Technology, China Reconstructs Magazine, Beijing. 1983.

Choain, Jean. "George Soulié de Morant", Meridiens Nos. 43-44. pps. 13-31. 1978.

Christie, Anthony. *Chinese Mythology.* Peter Bedrick Books, New York. 1985.

Chu, David C. and Dorothy W. Chu. *The Principles of Chinese Acupuncture Medicine.* Life Sciences Medical Labs. 1975.

Chuang, Yu-Min-1. *Chinese Acupuncture.* Oriental Society, Hanover, NH. 1972.

Chuang, Yu-Min-2. *The Historical Development of Acupuncture.* Oriental Healing Arts Institute. Los Angeles. 1982.

Connelly, Dianne M. *Traditional Acupuncture: The Law of the Five Elements.* The Center for Traditional Acupuncture. Columbia, MD 1979.

Cook, Trevor, M. *Samuel Hahnemann.* Thorson's Wellingborough. 1981.

Covell, Alan Carter -1. *Ecstasy, Shamanism in Korea.* Hollym International Corp. Seoul, Korea. 1983.

Covell, Alan Carter -2. *Shamanist Folk Paintings.* Hollym International Corp. Seoul, Korea. 1984.

Covell, Jon Carter. *Korea's Cultural Roots.* Hollym International Corp. Seoul, Korea. 1981.

Crozier, Ralph C. "Traditional Medicine in Modern China: Social, Political and Cultural Aspects," in *Modern China and Traditional Chinese Medicine.* G.B. Risse (ed.) Charles C. Thomas, Springfield. 1973.

Dale, Ralph Alan and Yan Cheng. *Dictionary of Acupuncture.* Dialectic Publishing. North Miami Beach. 1993.

de La Fuÿe, Roger-1. *Traité D'Acupuncture.* Le François. Paris. 1956. (second edition)

de La Fuÿe, Roger-2. *L'Acupuncture Moderne Pratique.* Le François. Paris. 1972.

DeWoskin, Kenneth J. (trans.) *Doctors, Diviners and Magicians of Ancient China: Biographies of Fang-shih.* Columbia University Press. New York. 1983.

Duke, Marc. *Acupuncture.* Pyramid Books, New York. 1972.

Duron, A., Ch. Laville-Mery and J. Borsarello. *Bioénergétique et Médecine Chinoise,* Maisonneuve, Moulins lès Metz. 1976.

Eberhard, Wolfram. *A Dictionary of Chinese Symbols.* Routledge and Keegan Paul. London. 1986.

Eckman, Peter-1. "Acupuncture and Science", Internat. J. Chin. Med. Vol. 1, No. 1, March 1984. pps. 3-8.

Eckman, Peter-2. *The Book of Changes in Traditional Oriental Medicine.* Traditional Acupuncture Institute. Columbia, MD. 1987.

Essentials of Chinese Acupuncture. Foreign Languages Press. Beijing. 1980.

Faubert, André. *Traité didactique d'Acupuncture Traditionelle.* Editions de la Maisnie. Paris. 1977.

Feng Yu Lan (trans.) *Chuang-Tzu.* Foreign Languages Press. Beijing. 1989.

Ferreyroles, Paul. *L'Acupuncture Chinoise.* Editions S.L.E.L. Lille. 1953.

Firebrace, Peter. "Review of Traditional Acupuncture, Vol. 2 by J.R. Worsley", Trad. Acup. Soc. J. (U.K.) No. 9, pps. 48-49, April, 1991.

Flaws, Bob-1. *Blue Poppy Essays.* Blue Poppy Press. Boulder. 1988.

Flaws, Bob-2. "Four LA Blocks to Therapy and TCM" Trad. Acup. Soc. J. (U.K.) No. 6, pps. 5-7, Nov. 1989.

Flaws, Bob-3. Preface to *Master Hua's Classic of the Central Viscera* by Yang Shou-zhong. Blue Poppy Press. Boulder. 1993.

Flaws, Bob, Charles Chase and Michael Helme. *Timing and the Times.* Blue Poppy Press. Boulder. 1986.

Footsteps of Yanagiya Sorei. Masako Yanagiya, editor. Ido No Nippon. Tokyo. 1964. (In Japanese)

Fox, Charles. Unpublished typescript and audiotape of an interview with J.R. Worsley on March 13, 1978. Author's collection.

Fu Shi yuan. "Present situation of Chinese Acupuncture and Moxibustion education and its prospective strategy". J. Trad. Chin. Med. (China) Vol 10, No. 1. pps. 3-5. 1990.

Fujikawa, Y. *Japanese Medicine.* Paul B. Hoeber. New York. 1934.

Fukushima, Kodo. *Meridian Therapy.* Toyo Hari Medical Association. Tokyo. 1991.

Fung Yu-Lan (trans.) *Chuang-Tzu.* Foreign Languages Press. Beijing. 1989.

Gaier, Harald. *Thorson's Encyclopaedic Dictionary of Homoeopathy.* Thorsons. London. 1991.

Girardot, N.J. *Myth and Meaning in Early Taoism.* University of California Press. Berkeley. 1983.

Gunji, Ryoichi. *Introduction to Simple Ryodoraku - Treatment.* Bunkodo. Tokyo. 1971.

Hammer, Leon. *Dragon Rises, Red Bird Flies.* Station Hill Press. Barrytown, NY. 1990.

Hashimoto, Masae. *Entry Gate to Moxibustion.* Shufu to Seikatsu Sha. Tokyo. 1964. (In Japanese)

Hashimoto, M. *Japanese Acupuncture.* P. Chancellor (ed.). Liveright. New York. 1966.

Hicks, John. "What is Five Element Acupuncture?" J. Chin Med. (U.K.), No. 25, pps. 3-10. Sept. 1987.

Hoe, Jock. *China From Earliest Times to 1840.* Peoples Republic of China. 1983.

Hoizey, Dominique and Marie-Joseph Hoizey. *A History of Chinese Medicine.* Edinburgh University Press. 1993.

Honma, Shohaku. *Keiraku Chiryo Kowa.* (Discourse on Meridian Therapy). Ido No Nippon. Yokosuka. 1949. (In Japanese).

Hsia, Emil C., Ilza Veith and Robert H. Geertsma (trans). *The Essentials of Medicine in Ancient China and Japan, Yasuyori Tamba's Ishimpo.* E.J. Brill. Leiden. 1986.

Hsu, Hong-Yen and William G. Peacher. *Chen's History of Chinese Medical Science.* Oriental Healing Arts Institute. 1977.

Huang-fu Mi. *The Systematic Classic of Acupuncture & Moxibustion.* Yang, S.Z. and Chace, C. translators. Blue Poppy Press. Boulder. 1994.

Huard, Pierre and Ming Wong -1. *La Médecine Chinoise Au Cours Des Siècles.* Les Editions Roger Da Costa. Paris. 1959.

Huard, Pierre and Ming Wong-2. *Chinese Medicine.* McGraw Hill. New York. 1968.

Huard, Pierre, Zensetsou Ohya and Ming Wong. *La Médecine Japonaise Des Origines A Nos Jours*. Les Editions Roger Da Costa. Paris. 1974.

Hucker, Charles O. *China's Imperial Past*. Stanford University Press. Stanford. 1975.

Hume, Edward H. *The Chinese Way in Medicine*. The Johns Hopkins Press. Baltimore. 1940.

Hyatt, Richard. *Chinese Herbal Medicine*. Schocken Books. New York. 1978.

Jacquemin, Jenine. "George Soulié de Morant, sa vie, son oeuvre". Rev. Française D'Acup. No. 42. pps. 9-31. 1985.

Jarricot, Henri and Ming Wong. "Essai sur l'Histoire de l'Acuponcture Chinoise" in *Nouveau Traité D'Acupuncture* by J.E.H. Niboyet. Maisonneuve. Paris. 1979.

Jayasuria, Anton. *Acupuncture Science*. Acupuncture Foundation of Sri Lanka. Columbo. 1981.

Jiang Yijun. "Clinical Application of the Crossing Points of Eight Extra Channels". J. Trad. Chin. Med. (China) Vol. 4. No. 1. pps. 77-82. March, 1984.

Kajdos, Vaclav. "The Akabane Method and its Application in Acupuncture." Am. J. Ac. Vol. 2. No. 4. pps. 266-271. Dec. 1974.

Kaltenmark, Max. *Lao Tzu and Taoism*. Stanford University Press. Stanford. 1969.

Kaptchuk, Ted-1. *The Web That Has No Weaver*. Congdon and Weed. N.Y. 1983.

Kaptchuk, Ted-2. Introduction to *Fundamentals of Chinese Medicine*. N. Wiseman and A. Ellis (trans.). Paradigm Publications. Brookline. 1985.

Kaptchuk, Ted, Giovanni Maciocia, Felicity Moir and Peter Deadman. "Acupuncture in the West". J. Chin. Med. (U.K.) No. 17. pps. 22-31. Jan. 1985.

Kespi, Jean-Marc. *Acupuncture*. Maisonneuve. Moulins lès Metz. 1982. (In French).

Kim Bong Han. "On the Meridian System". Journal of D.P.R.K. Acad. Med. Sci. 1963. (In Korean).

Kim, Dok Ho. *Acupuncture and Moxibustion*. Research Institute of Oriental Medicine. Seoul. 1987.

Kotzsch, Ronald E. -1. "Georges Ohsawa and the Japanese Religious Tradition". Doctoral Thesis. Harvard University. Cambridge. 1981.

Kotzsch, Ronald E.-2. *Macrobiotics Yesterday and Today*. Japan Publications. New York. 1985.

Kuon, Dowon -1. "A Study of Constitution Acupuncture". J. Internat. Cong. Acup. Mox. Japan Acup. Mox. Soc. pps. 149-167. 1965.

Kuon, Dowon -2. "Studies on Constitution - Acupuncture Therapy". Korean Central J. Med., Vol. 25. No. 3. pps. 327-342. Sept. 1973.

Kushi, Michio. *Acupuncture, Ancient and Future Worlds*. Tao Publications. Boston. 1973.

Kutchins, Stuart and Peter Eckman. *Closing the Circle: Lectures on the Unity of Traditional Oriental Medicine*. Shen Foundation. Fairfax, CA 1983.

Larre, Claude and Elisabeth Rochat de la Vallée-1. *Chinese Medicine From the Classics*. A series published by Monkey Press. Cambridge.

Larre, Claude and Elisabeth Rochat de la Vallée-2. *The Secret Treatise of the Spiritual Orchid*. Foreword by P. Eckman. Monkey Press. Cambridge. 1992.

Larre, Claude, Jean Schatz and Elisabeth Rochat de la Vallée. *Survey of Traditional Chinese Medicine*. (S. Stang trans.). Traditional Acupuncture Foundation. Columbia. 1986. (original French edition, 1979).

Lavier, Jacques A. -1. *Les bases traditionelles de l'Acupuncture Chinoise.* Maloine. Paris. 1964.

Lavier, Jacques A. -2. *Points of Chinese Acupuncture.* (P. Chancellor trans. and ed.). Health Science Press. Bradford. 1965.

Lavier, Jacques A. -3. *Histoire, doctrine et pratique de l'acupuncture chinoise.* Tchou. Paris. 1966.

Lavier, Jacques A. -4. *Vade-Mecum D'Acupuncture Symptomatique.* Maloine. Paris. 1968.

Lavier, Jacques A. -5. *Le Livre de la Terre et du Ciel, les secrets du Yi King.* Tchou. Paris. 1969.

Lavier, Jacques A. -6. *Bio-Energetique Chinoise.* Maloine. Paris. 1976.

Lavier, Jacques A. -7. (trans.) *Nei Tching Sou Wen.* Pardès. Puiseaux. 1990.

Lawson-Wood, Denis. *Chinese System of Healing.* Health Sciences Press. Greyshott. 1959. Foreword by Leslie Korth.

Lawson-Wood, Denis and Joyce Lawson-Wood -1. *Glowing Health Through Diet and Posture.* Health Science Press. Bradford. 1961.

Lawson-Wood, Denis and Joyce Lawson-Wood -2. *First Aid at Your Fingertips.* Health Science Press. Bradford. 1963.

Lawson-Wood, Denis and Joyce Lawson-Wood -3. *Acupuncture Handbook.* Health Science Press. Bradford. 1964.

Lawson-Wood, Denis and Joyce Lawson-Wood -4. *The Five Elements of Acupuncture and Chinese Massage.* Health Science Press. Bradford. 1965.

Lawson-Wood, Denis and Joyce Lawson-Wood -5. *The Incredible Healing Needles.* Samuel Weiser. New York. 1974.

Lawson-Wood, Denis and Joyce Lawson-Wood -6. *Judo Revival Points.* Health Science Press. Bradford. 1960. Revised edition published as *Acupuncture Vitality and Revival Points.* 1975.

Lawson-Wood, Denis and Joyce Lawson-Wood -7. *Progressive Vitality and Dynamic Posture.* Health Science Press. Bradford. 1977.

Lee, Johng Kyu and Sang Kook Bae. *Korean Acupuncture.* Ko Mun Sa. Seoul. 1974.

Lee, Miriam. *Master Tong's Acupuncture.* Blue Poppy Press. Boulder. 1992.

Legge, James (trans.). *The Texts of Taoism.* Dover Publications. NY. 1962.

Leung, Kok-Yuen. "The Five Yu in Classical Acupuncture". Am. J. Acup. Vol. 1. No. 4. pps. 151-167. 1973.

Levenson, Joseph R. and Franz Schurmann. *China: An Interpretive History.* University of California Press. Berkeley. 1969.

Lewith, George T. *Acupuncture— Its Place in Western Medical Science.* Thorsons. Wellingborough. 1982.

Li Yan. *Yi Xue Ru Men* (YXRM)-*The Basics of Medical Studies.* 1575. In Chinese.

Liaw Luying. *The Historical Outline of Acupuncture.* Unpublished manuscript in progress.

Liu, Da-1. *The Tao and Chinese Culture.* Schocken Books. New York. 1979.

Liu, Da-2. *I Ching Numerology.* Harper and Row. New York. 1979.

Liu, Frank and Liu Yan Mau. *Chinese Medical Terminology.* The Commercial Press. Hong Kong. 1980.

Liu Yanchi. *The Essential Book of Traditional Chinese Medicine.* Written and edited in collaboration with Kathleen Vian and Peter Eckman. Columbia University Press. 1988.

Low, Royston. *The Secondary Vessels of Acupuncture*. Thorsons. Wellingborough. 1983.

Lu, Gwei-Djen and Joseph Needham. *Celestial Lancets*. Cambridge University Press. Cambridge. 1980.

Lu, Henry C. -1. (trans.) *The Yellow Emperor's Classic of Internal Medicine and the Difficult Classic*. Academy of Oriental Heritage. Vancouver. 1978.

Lu, Henry C. -2. *Introduction to Chinese Classics in Medicine*. The Academy of Oriental Heritage. Vancouver. 1980.

Ma Kan-Wen. "The Roots and Development of Chinese Acupuncture: from Pre-history to Early 20th Century". J. Brit. Med. Acup. Soc. Vol. X. Supplement. 1992.

Maciocia, Giovanni -1. "History of Acupuncture". J. Chin. Med. (U.K.) No. 9. pps. 9-15. April, 1982.

Maciocia, Giovanni -2. *Tongue Diagnosis in Chinese Medicine*. Eastland Press. Seattle. 1987.

Manaka, Yoshio and Ian Urquhart. *The Layman's Guide to Acupuncture*. Weatherhill. New York. 1972. Foreward by Sally Reston.

Mann, Felix -1. *Acupuncture, The Ancient Chinese Art of Healing*. William Heinemann. London. 1962.

Mann, Felix -2. *The Treatment of Disease by Acupuncture*. William Heinemann Books. London. 1963.

Mann, Felix -3. *The Meridians of Acupuncture*. William Heinemann Books. London. 1964.

Mann, Felix -4. *Acupuncture: Cure of Many Diseases*. William Heinemann Books. London. 1971.

Mann, Felix -5. *Scientific Aspects of Acupuncture*. William Heinemann Books. London. 1983.

Mann, Felix -6. *Textbook of Acupuncture*. Heinemann Medical Books. Oxford. 1987.

Maspero, Henri. *Taoism and Chinese Religion*. University of Massachusetts Press. Amherst. 1981.

Matsumoto, Kiiko and Stephen Birch. *Five Elements and Ten Stems*. Paradigm Publications. undated.

McGavack, Thomas. *The Homeopathic Principle in Therapeutics*. Boericke & Tafel. Philadelphia. 1932.

Merton, Thomas. *The Way of Chuang Tzu*. New Directions. NY. 1965.

Mole, Peter. *Acupuncture, Energy Balancing For Body, Mind and Spirit*. Element Books. Shaftsbury. 1992.

Monnier, R. "L'Acupuncture des Années 1960 en Europe". La Revue Française de Médecine Traditionelle Chinoise. Vol. 133. pps. 49-51. 1989.

Morse, William R -1. *The Three Crosses in the Purple Mists*. Mission Book Co. Shanghai. 1928.

Morse, William R -2. "The Practices and Principles of Chinese Medicine". J. of West China Border Research Soc. Vol. 3. 1926 - 1929.

Morse, William R -3. *Chinese Medicine*. Paul B. Hoeber. New York. 1938.

Muramoto, Naboru. *Healing Ourselves*. Avon Books. New York. 1973. Compiled by Michel Abehsera.

Mussat, Maurice. *Acupuncture*. Médecine et Sciences Internationales. Paris. 1980. (In French)

Na, Chi. "General Concepts of the Pen-Tsao (The Chinese Herbals)". Bulletin of the Oriental Healing Arts Institute. Volume 5. No. 1. 1980.

NACA - North American College of Acupuncture. *Chinese Medical Philosophy and Principles of Diagnosis.* undated.

Nakatani, Yoshio and Kumio Yamashita. *Ryodoraku Acupuncture.* Ryodoraku Research Institute. Osaka. 1977.

Nakayama, T. *Acupuncture et Médecine Chinoise Vérifiées au Japon,* T. Sakurazawa and G. Soulié de Morant (trans). Le François. Paris. 1934.

National Symposia of Acupuncture and Moxibustion and Acupuncture Anaesthesia. Beijing. 1979.

Needham, Joseph. *Science and Civilization in China.* Vol. 2. Cambridge University Press. 1956.

Ni, Hua Ching. *The Book of Changes.* College of Tao. Los Anges. 1983.

Ni, Maoshing. *The Yellow Emoeror's Classic of Medicine* (translation and adaptation). Shambhala. Boston. 1995.

Niboyet, J.E.H. -1. *Essai sur L'Acupuncture Chinoise Pratique.* Editions Dominique Wapler. Paris. 1951.

Niboyet, J.E.H. -2. *Compléments D'Acupuncture.* Editions Dominique Wapler. Paris. 1955.

Niboyet, J.E.H. -3. "A propos de quelques propriétés électriques des points cutanés utilisés en Acupuncture." Actes des IVe Journées Internationales d'Acupuncture. pps. 87-89. 1959.

Niboyet, J.E.H. -4. *Le Traitement Des Algies Par L'Acupuncture.* Editions Jacques Lafitte. Paris. 1959.

Niboyet, J.E.H. -5. *Nouveau Traité D'Acupuncture.* Maisonneuve. Paris. 1979.

Obaidey, Edward. "Misao Takenouchi, Glimpses of an Eminent Acupuncturist". Pacific J. of Oriental Med. No. 3. 1994. pp.7-10.

O'Connor, John and Dan Bensky. (trans. and eds.) *Acupuncture, A Comprehensive Text.* Eastland Press. Chicago. 1981.

Ohsawa, Georges -1. *L'Acupuncture et la Médecine d'Extrême Orient.* Vrin. Paris. 1969. Preface by Dr. Chamfrault (1967).

Ohsawa, Georges -2. *Acupuncture and the Philosophy of the Far East.* Tao Books. Boston. 1973. B. Gardiner (trans. and ed.)

Ohsawa, Georges -3. *The Art of Peace.* GOMF. Oroville. 1990.

Otsuka Keisetsu. *30 Years of Kanpo.* Oriental Healing Arts Institute. Los Angeles. 1984.

Ozaki, Norman T. "Conceptual Changes in Japanese Medicine During the Tokugawa Period. Doctoral Thesis. UCSF. 1979.

Pálos, Stephan. *The Chinese Art of Healing.* Bantam Books. New York. 1971.

Peng Jingshan, "Seven Prescription and Ten Pharmaceutical Forms of Acupuncture and Moxibustion Therapy". Am. J. Ac. Vol. 14. No. 1. pps. 43-46. Jan. 1986.

Pennell, Rolla J. and Gordon D. Heuser. *The "How To" Seminar of Acupuncture for Physicians.* IPCI. Independence. 1973.

Porkert, Manfred. *The Theoretical Foundations of Chinese Medicine.* The MIT Press. Cambridge, MA. 1974.

Porter, Bill. *Road to Heaven, Encounters with Chinese Hermits.* Mercury House. San Francisco. 1993.

Qiu Mao-liang (ed.) *Chinese Acupuncture and Moxibustion.* Churchill Livingstone. Edinburgh. 1993.

Reader, Ian, Esben Andreasen and Finn Stefánsson. *Japanese Religions Past and Present*. Univ. of Hawaii Press. 1993.

Said, Hakim Mohammed. *Medicine in China*. Hamard Foundation. Karachi. 1981.

Scheffer, Mechthild. *Bach Flower Therapy*. Healing Arts Press. Rochester. 1988.

Schiffeler, John William. *The Legendary Creatures of the Shan Hai Ching*. Hwa Kang Press. Taipei. 1978.

Schipper, Kristofer. *The Taoist Body*. University of California Press. Berkeley. 1993. (original French edition, 1982)

Schmidt, Heribert -1. "Der Akabane Test". Deutsche Zeitschrift fuer Akupunktur. Vol. 13. No. 4. pps. 98-107. 1964.

Schmidt, Heribert -2. *Konstitutionelle Akupunktur*. Hippokrates Verlag. Stuttgart. 1988.

Schmidt, Josef M. "Die Geschichte der Akupunktur in Deutschland." Doctoral dissertation, University of Köln (in German). 1974.

Seem, Mark. "Beyond TCM Acupuncture: Treating the Energetic Core." Am J. Ac. Vol. 14. No. 4. pps. 363-367. Oct. 1986.

Shirota Bunshi. *Shinkyu Shinzui Sawado Ryu Ken Sho*. Ido No Nippon. 1941.

Shudo, Denmei. *Introduction to Meridian Therapy*. Eastland Press. Seattle. 1990.

Sivin, Nathan. *Traditional Medicine in Contemporary China*. Center for Chinese Studies. University of Michigan. Ann Arbor. 1987.

Small, Tolbert. "Acupuncture Anesthesia: A Review". Am. J. Ac. Vol. 2. No. 3. pps. 147-163. July, 1974.

So, James Tin Yau -1. *The Book of Acupuncture Points*. Paradigm Publications. Brookline. 1985.

So, James Tin Yau -2. *Treatment of Disease with Acupuncture*. Paradigm Publications. Brookline. 1987.

Song Tian Bin. *Atlas of the Tongue and Lingual Coatings in Chinese Medecine*. Editions Sinomedic. Boersch. (France). 1986.

Soulié de Morant, George -1. *Précis de la vrai Acuponcture chinoise*. Mercure de France. Paris. 1934.

Soulié de Morant, George -2. *L'Acuponcture Chinoise*. Maloine. Paris. 1972. (Tome 1, 2 originally published by Mercure de France, 1939 - 1941.)

Soulié de Morant, George -3. *Le Diagnostic par les pouls radiaux*. La Maisnie. 1983.

Soulie de Morant, George-4. *Chinese Acupuncture*. Paradigm Publications. Brookline. 1994.

Soulié de Morant, George and Paul Ferreyroles. "L'Acuponcture en Chine, vingt siècles av. J.C. et la Réflexothérapie moderne." L'Homéopathie Française, juin 1929.

Steiner, Stan. *Fusang, The Chinese Who Built America*. Harper and Row. New York. 1979.

Stiefvater, Eric H.W.-1 *Akupunktur als Neuraltherapie*. Haug Verlag. Ulm. 1953. (in German).

Stiefvater, Eric H.W.-2 *What is Acupuncture? How Does it Work?* Health Science Press. Bradford. 1971. (second edition, translated and edited by Leslie Korth) Original German edition, 1955. First English edition, 1962.

Stux, Gabriel and Bruce Pomeranz. *Acupuncture Textbook and Atlas*. Springer-Verlag. Berlin. 1987.

Sugiyama, Waichi. *Sugiyama's Complete Works*. Yoshida Kodo. Tokyo. 1932. (In Japanese).

Szuma Chien. *Records of the Historian.* Foreign Languages Press. Beijing. 1979.

Tany, Michio. "New Analgesia Technique Based on the Acupuncture Meridian Phenomenon." Am. J. Ac. Vol. 1. No. 4. pps. 203-209. 1973.

Tim, Wei Thiong Chan Wai. "George Soulié de Morant", Meridiens. No. 79. pps 14-125. 1987.

Tsui Chieh. *The Theory and Practice Concerning Methods of Supplement and Diminution.* (in Chinese) World Medicine Publisher. Taiwan. 1962.

Unschuld, Paul U. -1. *Medicine in China, A History of Ideas.* University of California Press. Berkeley. 1985.

Unschuld, Paul U. -2. "The Role of Traditional Chinese Medicine in Contemporary Health Care" in Proc. Symp. 9 and Satellite Symp. 8 of 17th International Congress Internal Medecine. Excerpta Medica. Amsterdam. 1985.

Unschuld, Paul U. -3. *Medicine in China, a History of Pharmaceutics.* University of California Press. Berkeley. 1986.

Unschuld, Paul U. -4. (trans) *Nan-Ching, The Classic of Difficult Issues.* University of California Press. Berkeley. 1986.

Van Nghi, Nguyen and M. Emmanuel Picou. *Pathogénie et Pathologie Energétiques en Médecine Chinoise.* Ecole Technique Don Bosco. Marseille. 1971 (2nd edition) Foreword by Lok Yee kung.

Veith, Ilza (trans) *The Yellow Emperor's Classic of Internal Medicine.* University of California Press. Berkeley. 1966.

Waldron, Arthur. *The Great Wall of China.* Cambridge University Press. Cambridge. 1990.

Waley, Arthur. *Three Ways of Thought in Ancient China.* Stanford University Press. Stanford. 1982.

Wallacker, Benjamin E. *The Huai-Nan-Tzu, Book Eleven: Behavior, Culture and the Cosmos.* American Oriental Society. New Haven. 1962.

Wallnofer, Heinrich and Anna Von Rottauscher. *Chinese Folk Medicine and Acupuncture.* Bell Publishing Co., New Yorl. 1965.

Wang Xuetai-1. "An Introduction to the Study of Acupuncture and Moxibustion in China (Part 1)". J. Trad. Chin. Med. (China) Vol. 4 No. 2. pps. 85-90. June, 1984.

Wang Xuetai-2. "Academic Achievements of Chinese Acupuncture and Moxibustion in Ancient and Modern Times" in Proc. Symp. 9 and Satellite Symp. 8 of 17th Internat. Cong. Int. Med., Excerpta Medica. Amsterdam, 1985.

Watson, Burton (trans.) *Cold Mountain.* Shambhala. Boston. 1992.

Weeks, Nora. *The Medical Discoveries of Edward Bach, Physician.* Keats. New Caanan. 1973.

Wieger, L. *Chinese Characters.* Dover Publications. New York. 1965.

Wilhelm, Richard and Cary F. Baynes (trans.) *The I Ching or Book of Changes.* Princeton University Press. Princeton. 1977.

Wong, Ed-1. *Chinese Acupuncture, Symptomatic Treatment.* No listing of author, publisher or date. Verified by Ralph Luciani, D.O.

Wong, Ed-2. *Chinese Acupuncture, A.P.P. Basic Seminar Study Manual No. 2.* No listing of author, publisher or date. Verified by Ralph Luciani, D.O.

Wong, Ed-3. *What is Acupuncture?,* a promotional brochure for A.P.P. Technique Seminars. No listing of author or date. Verified by Jim Shores.

Wong, K. Chimin and Wu Lien-Teh. *History of Chinese Medicine.* National Quarantine Service. Shanghai. 1936.

Worsley, J.R.-1. *Acupuncturists Therapeutic Pocketbook.* Publisher and date unknown.

Worsley, J.R.-2. *Traditional Chinese Acupuncture. Volume I. Meridians and Points.* Element Books. Tisbury. 1982.

Worsley, J.R.-3. *Traditional Acupuncture Volume II Traditional Diagnosis.* The College of Traditional Acupuncture. U.K. Leamington Spa. 1990.

Worsley, J.R.-4. *Is Acupuncture For You?* Harper and Row. New York. 1973.

Worsley, J.R.-5. *Is Acupuncture For You?* Revised Edition. Element books. Longmead. 1985.

Worsley, J.R. and M.H. Stemp. *The Case For Acupuncture.* Publisher unknown. First edition, 1967. Second edition undated. Foreword by Lok Yee Kung.

Worsley, John. "Professor J.R. Worsley, A Profile." Trad. Acup. Soc. J. No. 1. pps. 1-2. 1987.

Wu, K.C. *The Chinese Heritage.* Crown Publishers. New York. 1982.

Wu Wei-P'ing-1. *Chinese Acupuncture.* J. Lavier (trans. from Chinese) and P. Chancellor (trans. from French). Health Science Press. Denington Estate. 1962.

Wu Wei-P'ing-2. letter in Acup. Assn. Newsletter. (U.K.) Oct. 1966. pps. 6-7.

Xie Zhufan and Huang Xiaokai (eds) *Dictionary of Traditional Chinese Medicine.* The Commercial Press. Hong Kong. 1984.

Yang Ji-zhou. *Zhen Jiu Da Cheng* (ZJDC) - *Great Compendium of Acupuncture and Moxibustion.* 1601. In Chinese.

Yang Shou-zhong-1 (trans.) *Master Hua's Classic of the Central Viscera.* Blue Poppy Press. Boulder. 1993.

Yang Shou-zhong-2 (trans) *Li Dong-yuan's Treatise on the Spleen and Stomach,* Blue Poppy Press. Boulder. 1993.

Yoo Tae-woo. *Koryo Hand Acupuncture: Vol. 1.* P. Eckman (ed), Eum Yang Mek Jin. Seoul. 1988.

Zhang Zhongjing-1. *Shang Han Lun.* Translated and edited by H.Y. Hsu and W. Peacher. Oriental Healing Arts Institute. Los Angeles. 1981.

Zhang Zhongjing-2. *Chin Kuei Yao Lueh.* Translated and edited by H.Y. Hsu and S.Y. Wang. Oriental Healing Arts Institute. Los Angeles. 1983.

Zhang Zhongjing-3. *Treatise on Febrile Diseases Caused by Cold.* New World Press. Beijing. 1986.

Zhang Zhongjing-4. *Synopsis of Prescriptions of the Golden Chamber.* New World Press. Beijing. 1987.

Zhu Lian. *New Acupuncture.* Public Health Press. Beijing. 1955. (In Chinese)

INDEX

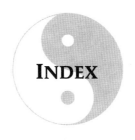